PRAISE FOR *MODERN INTEGRATIVE COUNSELING AND PSYCHOTHERAPY: A STEP-BY-STEP APPROACH*

"Bishop's step-by-step guide could be used daily by newer psychotherapists, and as a trustworthy handbook by seasoned ones. As psychotherapy grapples with the realization that we need to move beyond schools of psychotherapy, specific guidance about how to do so has been scarce. Bishop takes up this challenge with a research- and principles-based guide that is oriented around the events that are likely to occur in almost every course of psychotherapy. The clinical examples, including dialogues showing a master clinician at work, illustrate options for addressing typical events, how to use a range of techniques, and how important scientific evidence from outside psychotherapy can be applied for the benefit of our clients. This book will help guide the way toward more integrative psychotherapy."

—Tom Horvath, PhD, ABPP, president, Practical Recovery, California

"Whether you are at the beginning of your career as a therapist or possess extensive clinical experience, this book holds the potential to answer the leitmotif question 'What should I do next to help my clients in overcoming the challenges they face?' Dr. F. Michler Bishop presents us with a compendium that encompasses the most relevant therapy approaches, alongside an extensive collection of scientifically validated strategies. These resources can guide us in creating a personalized intervention plan. This book not only equips us with tools to aid our clients but also offers some practical self-care tips throughout this process. This is remarkable because, as therapists, we often become overly absorbed in our clients' issues. *Modern Integrative Counseling and Psychotherapy: A Step-by-Step Approach* is a valuable book that astonishes me with the complexity of the approach, the clarity of the writing, and the captivating way in which it is written."

—Petronela Predatu, clinical psychologist and psychotherapist, Romania; PhD student, Babeş-Bolyai University, Cluj-Napoca

"This book is a dream come true. It is an honest and open conversation with an experienced therapist who generously shares with you his secrets and life hacks. It gives you the most important information for practice and answers the questions you wanted to ask but have been afraid to: about self-disclosure, spirituality, medications, and integration techniques and models. For beginners, this book is a time and money saver because it provides the cornerstones for practice. For experienced therapists, it offers a fresh perspective on practicing therapy and new ways to improve."

—Dimitri Frolov, MD, psychologist and psychotherapist, formerly based in Moscow, Russia

"Dr. Bishop's book is quite refreshing. He highlights the importance of activities beyond therapy that can enhance someone's progress. His experience goes beyond the evidence, focusing on individual nuances."

—John C. Gramuglia, MBA, LICSW, MLADC, CPT; psychotherapist/personal trainer, The Villages, Florida

"I haven't encountered a book like this in my 50-plus years of studying and practicing psychology! It's as though I was sitting in a comfortable spot, listening to wisdom born of wide study and long practice being spoken from the heart as directly and casually as one speaks to a good friend about things that really matter. With the voice of a seasoned, insightful, compassionate practitioner, Dr. Bishop openly states his aim, ' . . . to help clients get back on track using a combination of activities, some of which are evidence-based, but some of which are not, at least not yet.' If you think you, or your students, could profit from such an experience, this book provides the opportunity."

—Hank Robb, PhD, ABPP, fellow, Association of Contextual Behavioral Science; private practice, Portland, Oregon

"Dr. Bishop has done it again. His wisdom and ability to weave the science and the application is exemplified in *Modern Integrative Counseling and Psychotherapy: A Step-by-Step Approach*. It is a must-read for early career professionals as it is full of guidance as practitioners are beginning their journey. And it is an excellent resource for seasoned practitioners as it reinforces best practices and ignites new applications. I am grateful this book exists as it makes practitioners a stronger resource to help those we serve. Thank you, Dr. Bishop!"

—Scott B. Goldman, PhD, performance psychologist, Golden State Warriors

"*Modern Integrative Counseling and Psychotherapy: A Step-by Step Approach* will be invaluable to early clinicians as well as seasoned clinicians who adopt an integrative approach to therapy. Drawing from years of experience, research, and a quest to find the best treatment for his clients, Dr. F. Michler Bishop provides a cogent and practical framework for integrating different schools of psychotherapy to meet clients' unique needs. He provides highly insightful and informative case examples alongside a clear, user-friendly guide for each phase of therapy. What an amazing resource this book is!"

—Candice R. S. Woo, PhD, private practice, New York, New York

"Consider this a guidebook to becoming an effective therapist if you're new to the field or becoming a more effective, well-rounded therapist if you've been practicing for some time. I've known Michler Bishop for nearly 30 years, and he is one of the most thoughtful and well-respected clinicians that I have had the privilege to know. I highly recommend *Modern Integrative Counseling and Psychotherapy* to practitioners regardless of their theoretical 'school' and training."

—Reid K. Hester, PhD, clinical psychologist; fellow, APA Addictions Division

"This book provides a remarkably well-integrated perspective on the classic and modern approaches of psychotherapy and counseling. This is further strengthened by the great organization of the techniques and tools used at each step of the intervention process."

—Oana A. David, PhD, Babeş-Bolyai University, Cluj-Napoca; director, Babeş-Bolai-PsyTech Psychology Clinic; chief editor, *Journal of Evidence-Based Psychotherapies*

"In France, we need F. Michler Bishop! All French practitioners should read this complete and great book about integrative treatments. Instead of a general model, Dr. Bishop understands that seven billion people, when they are psychologically disturbed, need seven billion answers!"

—Didier Pleux, PhD, private practice, Paris, France

"This book opened my eyes to the advantages of taking techniques from all the therapeutic domains. I'm excited to adapt this approach in a collectivist culture and see its impact in Asian countries. It is an insightful and intriguing read and paves a new path in delivering therapy."

—Roshana Wickremaratchi, psychological well-being practitioner, Colombo, Sri Lanka

"This fantastic book examines the reasons many clinicians mistakenly rely on a single school of psychotherapy and proposes that integrating various therapeutic modalities provides the highest quality of client care. Bishop presents a step-by-step guide to the fundamentals of clinical care, from agenda setting and homework to ongoing assessment, and boldly tackles the gray areas in between. Using historical context, research studies, theory, and engaging anecdotes, this book is not only accessible and useful but also interesting and memorable, besides being very enjoyable to read. I have no doubt many graduate programs will adopt this as required reading, and those of us farther along will benefit from it as well."

**—J. Ryan Fuller, PhD, cofounder, My Best Practice;
executive director, New York Behavioral Health**

"This exceptional book will help clinicians apply the knowledge and criteria for selecting the best treatment possible and present a set of general and empirically supported principles from a variety of approaches that can be used as different treatment options. This easy-to-use book addresses many aspects of emotional problems with treatment strategies that match up with different client characteristics. As Dr. Bishops says, 'Humans are much more complex than any textbook or approach,' and this book can guide psychotherapists and counselors to add to their repertoire of techniques and help many more clients efficiently."

**—Hugo Galo, PhD, clinical psychologist and psychotherapist;
codirector, Instituto de Terapia Racional Emotiva, Lima, Peru**

"F. Michler Bishop's new book is a welcome addition to the field from a renowned senior practitioner in the field of cognitive behavior therapy, which, as we know, was one of the first supported by scientific evidence. Hearing him advocate for an integration of the best techniques from established therapies with other activities that the client has found helpful makes the book more credible. He has given much attention to detail in systematically outlining what clinicians might consider doing during each section of a semi-structured, six-part therapy session, including how to use between-session time effectively. He advocates for therapists to take into account the cultural context and to adopt a humble, curious, collaborative therapeutic stance rather than an authoritarian one, and to be open to not-knowing, leaving the onus or burden of proof to scientists and researchers to investigate the reason why something works. Therefore, this book is a welcome addition to both a college graduate's and a seasoned practitioner's library. I enjoyed reading it."

**—Karl DeSouza, MD, director and lead psychotherapist,
Listening Ear Counselling and Consultancy, Singapore**

"We all know how difficult it is to grasp those elements that make up a great therapist, a therapist who can deal with many different clients in terms of age, socioeconomic bracket, sexual orientation, and cultural background. F. Michler Bishop has written a very important book in which he integrates all those elements in a very practical way. The approach is built on the firm base of CBT, but also on new developments in the field of emotions and body work: mindfulness, imagery, yoga, and trauma work. It integrates research-based interventions and alternative healing procedures that work for a particular client. It looks so simple and clear that one wonders why this has not been written before."

—**Erik Jongman, psychotherapist, Amsterdam, Netherlands**

"This new book by F. Michler Bishop is not just another guide for effective therapy but an example of the creative integration of many types of modern cognitive behavioral therapy and other types of psychotherapy by an experienced practitioner. His half-century of experience has been combined into a coherent holistic approach. I highly recommend it to be read not only by beginners but also by experienced specialists in the field of psychology and psychotherapy to expand their view of the human phenomenon, the possibilities of therapy, and the ways of change provided by modern therapeutic technologies."

—**Dmitrii Kovpak, PhD, MD, North-Western State Medical University named after I. I. Mechnikov; president, Association for Cognitive Behavioral Psychotherapy of Russia; board member, International Association of Cognitive Behavioral Therapy**

"For some people in Latin America, especially in countries such as Peru, the belief that they can be truly cured through atypical or non-evidenced treatments is very real. Although it might be challenging not to question non-evidence-based beliefs, we can teach ourselves that listening, empathizing, and being present with clients of all religious beliefs and cultural backgrounds is foundational. A number of these beliefs can be protective factors. Dr. Bishop's book advocates for such a truly integrative approach, and for that reason, it will be very helpful to new as well as seasoned practitioners as a guide to work respectfully, collaboratively, and efficiently.

"This book reflects Dr. Bishop's years of experience as a clinician. Written in accessible language, it presents how therapists can structure an integrated approach to provide the best possible treatment for clients, move beyond specific schools of therapy, and consider step-by-step guiding principles. It is a must-read for therapists who want to work more efficiently and better help their clients today."

—**Natalia Ferrero, clinical psychologist; founder and director, Psicotrec Institute, Lima, Peru**

"This book is not just a manual—it's a kind of manifesto that asks the counselor in training to take seriously what can be learned across a wide range of methods, once most of the limitations of 'schools' are abandoned. Drawing from Bishop's extensive experience with addiction, mood disorders, and behavior change, this book provides a sure-footed step-by-step guide for addressing such issues as how to build a working relationship, set an agenda, enhance motivation, or foster acceptance, compassion, and change. In the process-based world of evidence-based psychotherapy that is upon us, these skills help build a foundation from which students across a wide range of orientations can begin to learn how to change the biopsychosocial processes that will uplift the lives they serve."

—**Steven C. Hayes, PhD, Foundation Professor of Psychology Emeritus, University of Nevada, Reno**

Modern Integrative Counseling and Psychotherapy

A Step-by-Step Approach

F. Michler Bishop, PhD

ROWMAN & LITTLEFIELD
Lanham • Boulder • New York • London

Acquisitions Editor: Lilith Dorko
Assistant Acquisitions Editor: Sarah Rinehart
Sales and Marketing Inquiries: textbooks@rowman.com

Published by Rowman & Littlefield
An imprint of The Rowman & Littlefield Publishing Group, Inc.
4501 Forbes Boulevard, Suite 200, Lanham, Maryland 20706
www.rowman.com

86-90 Paul Street, London EC2A 4NE

British Library Cataloguing in Publication Information Available

Library of Congress Cataloging-in-Publication Data

Names: Bishop, F. Michler, author.
Title: Modern integrative counseling and psychotherapy / F. Michler Bishop, PhD, Albert Ellis Institute.
Description: Lanham : Rowman & Littlefield, [2024] | Includes bibliographical references and index.
Identifiers: LCCN 2023038848 (print) | LCCN 2023038849 (ebook) | ISBN 9781538175590 (cloth) | ISBN 9781538175606 (paperback) | ISBN 9781538175613 (epub) Subjects: LCSH: Eclectic psychotherapy. | Psychotherapy—Methodology. | Evidence-based psychotherapy.
Classification: LCC RC489.E24 B57 2024 (print) | LCC RC489.E24 (ebook) | DDC 616.89/14—dc23/ eng/20231025
LC record available at https://lccn.loc.gov/2023038848
LC ebook record available at https://lccn.loc.gov/2023038849

This book is dedicated to
Lucas Michler Bishop
who helps make this a better world
and
to the memory of
Manik de Silva Wijeyeratne and Neela (Nangi) Gunatilleke
who both made this world a better place for many people despite many challenges

Contents

Acknowledgments   xi

Introduction   xiii

PART I: MODERN INTEGRATIVE COUNSELING AND PSYCHOTHERAPY   1

Chapter 1: Moving Beyond Schools of Psychotherapy   3

Chapter 2: Guiding Principles for Modern Integrated Counseling and Psychotherapy   7

PART II: INITIAL IN-SESSION AND BETWEEN-SESSION WORK: STEP-BY-STEP   17

Chapter 3: Step 1: Build the Working Relationship: Enhance Hope and Motivation   19

Chapter 4: Step 2: Initial Assessment   29

Chapter 5: Step 3: Agree on the Therapeutic Goals   39

Chapter 6: Step 4: Set the Agenda   47

Chapter 7: Step 5: In-Session Work   49

Chapter 8: Step 6: Agree on Between-Session Work   61

Chapter 9: Working with Diverse Clients   71

PART III: SUBSEQUENT SESSIONS   79

Chapter 10: Ongoing Assessment, Evaluating Between-Session Work, Checking on Therapeutic Goals, and Setting the Agenda   81

Chapter 11: Facilitating Acceptance, Compassion, and Change: Mindfulness and Metastability   87

Chapter 12: Facilitating Acceptance, Compassion, and Change: Emotion-Focused and Imagery-Focused Work   97

Chapter 13: Facilitating Acceptance, Compassion, and Change: Genetics, Neurochemistry, and Neuroplasticity   109

Chapter 14: Moving Forward, Sliding Back: Managing Change and Metastability   117

Chapter 15: If Needed, Dig Deeper: Past-Focused Work, Trauma, and Childhood
    Issues   123

Chapter 16: Subsequent Between-Session Exercises   135

PART IV: OTHER ISSUES   143

Chapter 17: Self/Selves, Identity/Identities, and Change   145

Chapter 18: Integrating Coaching   157

Chapter 19: Medications: Are They Right for Your Client?   163

Chapter 20: Build Your Practice, Protect Yourself, and Prevent Burnout   173

References   185

Index   197

About the Author   207

Acknowledgments

Having been affected by my reading of multicultural literature and by the ongoing influence of my mentor at the College at Old Westbury, Dr. Charshee McIntyre, I first must acknowledge the people who came before me, especially the ones who have inspired me throughout my life. There are many from diverse cultures and countries and socioeconomic groups, but two stand out. My great-aunt Lala, Ethel Clark, taught me that one could always try to do something no matter your age. When I was seven, during a visit to the American Museum of Natural History in New York City, she enthusiastically had the two of us sign up for a trip to the moon when that became possible. Despite no university education, she taught herself ancient Greek and Latin, as well as French and German, and, among other jobs, cataloged alchemy book collections.

My cousin, Storrs Myron Bishop III, "Bish," also taught me that you could often do what you dreamed of doing if you dared to try. He skied Tuckerman's Ravine (missing his graduation from college to do so), surveyed the DEW line in Alaska, became a parachuter with the 82nd Airborne, lovingly bullied me, always referring to me as "Bugs" (short for "Bugs Bunny") because of my buck teeth, and taught me how to hitchhike. He turned his back on a corporate job on the East Coast and went out west to work as, among other things, an outfitter, farmer, and rancher, raising cattle and Norwegian Fjord horses in Ennis, Montana. He was also very active in the local, state, and national boards of education.

Without Great-Aunt Lala's and Bish's inspirational examples, I might never have dared to do many of the things that I have done in my life. I am also grateful for the influence of many other people, especially my mother and father for their support, my loving sister, Margi, and my uncle Hamp Marsh, "Unc." In addition, I have been fortunate to have wonderful families in this country and Sri Lanka, including a kind sister-in-law, Nangi; many equally wonderful brothers-in-laws, Bill Maynard, my sister's husband, Nangi's husband, Amar Gunatilleke, and Lalith, Manik, Rony, Dilip and Harin de Silva Wijeyeratne; and the rest of my 36-strong DSW clan. In their own ways, they have all influenced my thinking and my life, and I am indeed grateful.

At the Institute, I learned and was influenced by many people that worked there or I met there, including Drs. Albert Ellis, Ray DiGiuseppe, Kristene Doyle, Didier Pleux, Hank Robb, Manolo Mas Baga, and Windy Dryden. And I want to thank members of the Psychology Department at Old Westbury, especially Drs. Fred Millan, Runi Mukherji, Lorenz Neuwirth, and Lisa Whitten for their support, and the late Charshee McIntyre and Makanda Ken McIntrye for their wise advice and guidance. I was also very fortunate to have been influenced by the work of many colleagues in psychology, including Drs. Carlo DiClemente, Tom Horvath, Scott Kellogg, Bruce Liese, Barbara McCrady, William Miller, Linda Sobell, Mark Sobell, Andrew

Tatarsky, Katie Witkiewitz, and the many, many other researchers and clinicians who, through their articles, chapters, books, and presentations enriched my professional life and affected the way I do therapy. Earlier in my life, I was also fortunate to have worked with Dr. Caleb Gattegno and Dr. Dennis Shulman, and in Spain, my good friends, the late Vicente Fayos and Pedro Roca, both influenced me in their own ways. Much earlier, Raul Schkolnik, from Santiago, Chile, and Havana, Cuba, Tony Deepe, Adirondack guide, and Elmer, the first mate that I worked under on the Mississippi River, also played a large role in the way I think and have tried to live.

I am also deeply grateful to my friends Dexter Coolidge, Tim Allen, Larry Arancio, Bart Chezar, Barbara Jaffess, Mervyn Keizer, Mary Kenny, David Miller, Monika Napoleon, David Rathbun, Vicki Wolfe, and the late Bob Fisk and Tim Huff for all that they have contributed to my life and my thinking and all the fun, wisdom, support, and friendship they have provided.

I also want to thank all the clients and group members over the years who have made me wiser and, I think, a better therapist.

Finally, without the enthusiasm and help of the Rowman & Littlefield team, especially Lilith Dorko, Sarah Rinehart, and Jenna Dutton, this book would not exist.

My children Tonya, Manena, David, Anusha, and Arun, and my grandchild, Lucas, have always been and continue to be an inspiration for me in more ways than they can imagine, for which I am very, very grateful. Finally, I thank my wife, Nelun de Silva Wijeyeratne, the love of my life and a rock of stability, especially during times of great difficulties and stress, and the spirit behind innumerable wonderful adventures and happy times.

Introduction

When I was in training and working with a client, Marie, I was stumped. Marie was employed as an administrator in the VA in New York City, but she was not moving up in her career. She felt, perhaps correctly, that the men in her office preferred to work with men and most of the time promoted men. A three-year relationship had ended, she was 34 and doubted she would ever meet anyone or ever get married, and she very much wanted children. She had been depressed once before when she was in college, but now she also suffered from intense bouts of anxiety and occasional panic attacks, and sometimes fits of rage.

Fortunately, when she once became suicidal, I did not feel petrified and alone, because I had a number of good supervisors for guidance and support, including Dr. Albert Ellis, the founder of the first form of cognitive behavioral therapy (CBT), rational emotive behavior therapy (REBT; Ellis, 1962; Ellis & Harper, 1979). As I was only a year into my two-year training, I was continually anxious. I was reading everything I could get ahold of and watching video-tapes of people doing therapy, but I was so unsure, always wondering, "Am I doing the right thing? What should I do now?"

Week after week nothing I tried to do seemed to help Marie very much. Because I was in training to do REBT, besides listening empathetically and taping each session for her and for me, I asked questions like, "What do you think you are telling yourself that might be making your depression worse?" or "What do you think contributes to making you so anxious?" She shared that she thought she would never succeed in business and that she might wind up "an old spinster, like my Aunt Anne."

We also did ABC(DE) exercises and inference chaining, which helped. And she went to a psychiatrist and started taking Prozac. But after two more months, she was still not making much progress, so I said, "I think you should try something else. Maybe learning a new form of yoga or tai chi might help." I suggested that she go online and look for something that might appeal to her, perhaps a retreat or a workshop at Kripalu or the Omega Institute, two places on the East Coast and in driving distance.

Marie chose a monastery in the Catskill mountains outside of New York City. It lets AA use its facilities for weekend retreats. She was also overdrinking at times. She had attended a few AA meetings but didn't feel comfortable there, but she wanted to have more control over her drinking or quit.

She went to the Catskills four different times during the next year as we continued to work together. She changed in many different ways. She had become more comfortable being asser-tive and started to look for a new job in a "more enlightened" (her term) company. She was no longer depressed and had not had a panic attack in over a year.

In our last session, after reminding her that I never "terminate" anyone (a terrible term and idea; see chapter 20) and that she could always call me for a "brush up session" or a "booster shot," I asked her what she thought had helped most, therapy, the medication, her between-session work, what?

"Sitting at 5:00 a.m. for an hour. I thought I was going to die the first time, but as you would say, 'And, look, you didn't die,'" she said with a big smile. "I learned so much at those retreats, about myself, about meditation, about tolerating other people."

Over the years, I have learned that clients benefit from all sorts of activities and techniques, some of them evidence based and some of them not. In the past 50 years, a revolution in psychotherapy has occurred. This book pulls together the various elements of that revolution. It is designed to provide beginning clinicians and those who want to improve what they are already doing with new ideas and help. I have written it as a guidebook for more effective therapy. I suggest ways to incorporate the best from (in alphabetical order), ACT, CBT, CPS, CT, DBT, EFT, IPT, MBCT, and REBT, as well as other effective schools of psychotherapy, including existential therapy, feminist therapy, and a variety of psychodynamic therapies, such as brief psychodynamic therapy.

How has psychotherapy changed in the past 50 years? There have been at least 10 significant changes: (1) Insight is no longer the primary process of change. The development of skills for emotional regulation, resilience, and distress tolerance has equal importance. (2) Therapy has become future oriented and goal directed. (3) Between-session work, sometimes referred to as "homework," has become almost as important as in-session work. (4) Therapy has become a collaborative endeavor. The therapist is not always assumed to know best. (5) The focus has shifted from curing pathology toward helping people live more fulfilling lives as the result of developments in mindfulness-based therapies and positive psychology. (6) Therapy sessions have become more structured. (7) Briefer therapy has become the norm. (8) Neuroscience and the popularity of the medical (brain disease) model have grown exponentially, as has research into the plasticity of the brain. (9) CBT and its many forms are currently used by the majority of therapists around the world. (10) But research has shown that other therapies work, as well.

In addition, over the past 10 years: (1) Clinicians and researchers have begun to take into account other factors, such as culture, systemic racism, and identity issues. (2) Mental health counselors, pastoral counselors, social workers, and psychiatric nurses have become the primary deliverers of mental and behavioral health services. (3) Self-help has continued to grow as a means of self-guided change with increasing use of websites, wearables, webinars, podcasts, and apps. (4) More attention is focused on behavioral problems, such as overeating, stress management, attention deficit and hyperactivity disorder (ADHD), and addictive behaviors. (5) Finally, a combination of strategies, techniques, and activities—some research based and some from other ways of healing—are usually necessary to effectively help clients manage or overcome their difficulties.

Psychological problems do not often change quickly, and they may occur on and off during a person's life. What may change, however, is the way someone responds. To manage such problems, clients have to learn and combine a variety of strategies, including, at times, medications. Dr. Elyn Saks, University of Southern California law professor and MacArthur Award winner, in a *New York Times* (2013) article shared that she uses 10 ways to manage her schizophrenia. Fortunately, most of our clients are not suffering from something as serious as schizophrenia, but they still may need to combine a variety of strategies to manage their difficulties.

As those of us who work as clinicians know, humans are much more complex than any textbook suggests, and they come into our offices with myriad, complex, interacting issues and mixed motivations. No one school of psychotherapy will help each and every one of them. An innovative, integrative, individualized approach must be employed. As suggested by Norcross and Wampold (2018), a unique therapy for each client must be created and adjusted and readjusted over time. I hope you will find this book useful for that purpose.

PART I

Modern Integrative Counseling and Psychotherapy

Chapter 1

Moving Beyond Schools of Psychotherapy

There are literally hundreds of schools of psychotherapy, including some of the better-known "brands" listed below:

1. Acceptance and Commitment Therapy (ACT)
2. Adlerian Therapy
3. Attachment-Based Therapy
4. Behavior Therapy (BT)
5. Behavioral Activation Therapy
6. Bioenergetics
7. Brief Psychodynamic Therapy
8. Brief Relational Therapy
9. Client-Centered Therapy
10. Cognitive Therapy (CT)
11. Cognitive Behavioral Therapy (CBT)
12. Cognitive Processing Therapy (CPT)
13. Compassion-Focused Therapy (CFT)
14. Cyclical Psychodynamic Psychotherapy
15. Deliberate Practice
16. Dialectical Behavior Therapy (DBT)
17. Emotion Focused Therapy (EFT)
18. Emotion Regulation Therapy (ERT)
19. Existential Psychotherapy
20. Exposure and Response Prevention (ERP)
21. Exposure-Based Cognitive Therapy (EBCT)
22. Eye Movement Desensitization and Reprocessing (EMDR)
23. Family Therapy
24. Feminist Therapy
25. Functional Analytic Psychotherapy (FAP)
26. Future-Directed Therapy (FDT)
27. Future-Oriented Therapy (FOT)
28. Gestalt Therapy
29. Graduated Exercise Therapy
30. Harm Reduction Psychotherapy
31. Humanistic Therapy
32. Integrative Therapy
33. Internal Family Systems (IFS)

34. Interpersonal Psychotherapy
35. Jungian Therapy
36. Lifetrack Therapy
37. Logotherapy
38. Mindfulness-Based Cognitive Therapy (MBCT)
39. Mindfulness-Based Stress Reduction (MBSR)
40. Motivational Enhancement Therapy (MET)
41. Motivational Interviewing (MI)
42. Multicultural Therapy, Cultural-Sensitive Therapy
43. Multimodal Therapy
44. Multisystemic Therapy
45. Narrative Therapy
46. Person-Centered Therapy
47. Positive Psychotherapy
48. Psychoanalysis
49. Psychodynamic Psychotherapy
50. Psychopharmacotherapy
51. Rational Emotive Behavior Therapy (REBT)
52. Reality Therapy
53. Relapse Prevention
54. Schema Therapy
55. Self-Examination Therapy
56. Self-System Psychotherapy
57. Solution-Focused Brief Therapy
58. Systemic Therapy
59. Transactional Analysis
60. Transdiagnostic CBT
61. Trauma Recovery and Empowerment Model
62. Unified Protocol

So many distinct schools of psychotherapy for a counselor or therapist to choose from! Past APA president Walter Mischel has named this the "toothbrush" problem. Everyone is in the same field, but no one wants to use someone else's toothbrush, that is, theory or approach. So, they create a new one. But, as he notes, "If building a cumulative science is the goal, one has to avoid parallel play or repackaging ideas and findings already available" (Mischel, 2008, n.p.). This book is designed to help you cut through the confusion and anxiety looking at such a list may cause.

There is a long history of efforts to integrate approaches to psychotherapy and counseling (Castonguay et al., 2015; Cody, 2018; Goldfried, 2019; Hofmann & Hayes, 2019; Norcross & Goldfried, 2005). Many practicing therapists and counselors, when asked what kind of therapy they practice, say, "eclectic," which often means some form of integrated care. However, usually they consciously or unconsciously believe in a core theory or school, and that has a major impact on the way they work. This usually reflects how they were trained. Broadly speaking, all practitioners work from one of four perspectives: psychodynamic, cognitive-behavioral, humanistic, or family systems. Working from their core system or their theoretical orientation, they then add techniques from the other three major orientations. They integrate or combine ways of working or interventions, perhaps using different names—techniques, strategies, processes, exercises—for what they actually do, which is primarily determined by what they think will be helpful to the unique individual sitting in front of them.

I am opposed to schools of psychotherapy. In this sense, I would prefer that psychotherapy become more like modern medicine, which has many techniques to help people with a wide variety of illnesses. A cardiologist chooses from a variety of treatment options—medications, pacemakers, stents, valve transplants, whole heart transplants—and discusses them with a patient. Those treatment options were not available to the cardiologist 50 years ago. The field of cardiology has completely changed. The same needs to happen in counseling and psychotherapy.

Why are schools of psychotherapy so popular? Schools—especially new schools—provide hope, much like new religions: This will work. This will provide effective help to those I want to help. New religions function much the same way and are currently the fastest-growing forms of religious practice on the planet. In addition, schools help therapists decide what to do and how to work in their office. If someone chooses to work with a clinician who practices a form of psychodynamic therapy, their therapy will look very different from what they would experience if they chose an ACT or MBCT or DBT therapist. But we now have the option of using an integrated, combined approach, the central goal of this book.

The development of a science of counseling and psychotherapy is the long-range goal, but there is no reason that we cannot broaden our scientific investigations to include other methods of healing psychological distress. Most of the forms of psychotherapy were created by white middle- or upper-class males, many of whom were nonreligious and some of whom were virulently anti-religious. Perhaps as a result, insufficient attention has been paid to what a client may have found useful in terms of techniques or rituals from their own culture or religion. To some extent the integration of mindfulness and meditation into modern counseling and psychotherapy is a good example of what can happen.

When I started in 1987, I decided to focus on addictions in addition to treating clients trying to manage their major depression, bipolar issues, anxiety, procrastination, and relationship issues. Addictions are right on the cusp of automatic, conditioned behaviors and intentional, thoughtful behaviors. Studying how to help people change addictive behaviors has helped me work more effectively with people grappling with other problems.

Over the past 30 years, I have worked with many people who want to change. They want to change how they feel and behave. Working together, we usually have to figure out three things: How to *start* certain behaviors. How to *stop* other behaviors. And how to *maintain* the ones my clients want. All of that is very behavioral, but how they *feel* about starting or stopping and maintaining a behavior often determines how difficult it is to change. Consequently, feelings, both emotional and physiological, are central in this book. Of course, what the clients are thinking is important, too, including what they imagine about starting, stopping, or maintaining a behavior. Finally, their values and goals play a key role. What do they want to do with their lives? What kind of person do they want to be?

Many novels and movies focus on people who do not change and who may create havoc for those around them. But they are not the norm. Even if people think that failure to change is thought to be the norm, it is not. Fortunately, many studies show that people change over time, often dramatically (Bishop, 2018; Miller, 2004; Roberts & Mroczek, 2008).

Modern Integrative Counseling and Psychotherapy is designed to help you practice better. It reflects the significant changes in therapy over the past 50 years. Many experienced clinicians already integrate a variety of techniques into their sessions, but for beginning counselors and therapists, it is difficult to know what to do from moment to moment in a session. For that reason, this book guides you step by step.

Textbox 1.1. Research Note #1: Is Staying Up on the Research Important?

I know that some of my friends who are clinicians never look at research. They do not feel it has any relevance for how they practice. They studied very hard to learn a particular way of working, and it has done well for them, so why look at the research? If you are content to use one approach with all of your clients, then I understand.

However, this seems a little bit like my cardiologist not keeping up on the research. I can tell from our conversations that that is not the case. He cites research for his suggestions. But he does not take a solely top-down model. He has more than 25 years of experience and he knows a great deal, but he offers me a menu of options. Ultimately, I choose from among those options, perhaps one but more probably a combination (e.g., medication and a pacemaker).

Since the 1950s, we have learned a great deal that is relevant for both cardiology and counseling and psychotherapy. Much of what is in this book would not have been included 70 years ago. It was not known, and it is the result of research.

Everyone was curious when they were 1 day old and 5 years old. Unfortunately, sometimes schools and teachers destroy the love of learning and curiosity in people. They may continue to be curious but only about the latest sale or what a celebrity or a politician is doing. When they think about something that might help their work, they're not so curious! They get anxious.

Schools and schooling may have made learning anxiety producing, but over the next 70 years, we will learn all sorts of useful, wonderful things that will help us help clients. If counselors and psychotherapists are not open to that, what a loss!

I have included boxes with research notes throughout the book as examples of some of the remarkable things that we have learned over the past 70 years. No doubt, many, many research studies are of no help to us as clinicians, but some are. It is part of our job to keep up on what is happening in our field. I assume and hope that my internist and cardiologist are doing so.

Chapter 2

Guiding Principles for Modern Integrated Counseling and Psychotherapy

One of the leaders in the movement to integrate psychotherapies, Dr. Marvin Goldfried, has suggested that practitioners from different schools of psychology could probably agree on some basic principles (Goldfried, 2019). Given a short list of such guiding principles, they could work with their client using various approaches, strategies, processes, interventions, or techniques based on their understanding of what might work best for that particular, individual client.

The following seven guiding principles underlie the way of working advocated in this book:

1. Build the relationship, hope, and motivation.
2. Respect the client's culture and be open to integrating alternative ways of healing.
3. Be future oriented and goal focused.
4. When needed, process the impact of the past.
5. Facilitate acceptance and change.
6. Collaboratively work with the client to find a combination of strategies and techniques that help.
7. Ultimately, it is the client who decides which combination of strategies and techniques to use.

Most modern therapists use empirically supported techniques, but research is fairly new in the field of psychotherapy—in the Western world, a little over 100 years old—and many ways of healing have not been studied. Some clients may have found other ways of healing very effective, so helping them to restart what has worked for them in the past is a critical element of modern counseling and psychotherapy.

A COMBINED, COLLABORATIVE APPROACH

In some instances, changing one factor contributing to a client's problem can have a significant impact. However, changing a combination of factors is often necessary. That is also true when someone gets the flu. They may rest more, drink more liquids, take Advil or something similar, and change the kind and quantity of food and liquids they consume (e.g., they abstain from alcohol or drink tea instead of coffee). In addition, over time, their immune system kicks in and begins to destroy the virus. It is the combination that works. Had they drunk alcohol excessively and not rested while they were ill, the results might have been different.

What combination of techniques differs significantly from person to person. For some, it may be a combination of specific techniques and/or activities (e.g., deep diaphragmatic breathing, insight into dysfunctional family relationships, singing in a choir, and learning a new language). For another, it may be a combination of some form of CBT, medication, meditation, a new and more secure job with better benefits, and getting out of a bad relationship. Ultimately, the client determines and learns what combination works best.

This book also advocates for a combined bottom-up, top-down, collaborative approach. The traditional medical model is a purely top-down model, as is psychoanalysis. The doctor knows best. Compliance is the key to getting better. Resistance can be a problem.

In a bottom-up approach, the client is the expert. They know themselves best. Compliance is not a part of this model and "resistance" is seen as being stuck. Clients want to change but can't seem to figure out how.

This approach builds on and combines both. The counselor or therapist, like a good athletic coach or a good medical doctor, has studied hard, has been around for a while, has paid attention and tried to make sense of what they have observed. They have experience and expertise, and that expertise can be drawn on to help. Clients, in turn, know a lot about themselves, but they may not have been able to connect the dots. Working together, a good clinician can help them figure out what is causing problems in their life and what is not, what helps them get unstuck and what does not, what helps them move forward and what does not, and what helps them have a more meaningful and enjoyable life, and what does not.

Given the complexity of each individual, what helps one person may harm another. This is true in the medical world, as well. Unfortunately, most research over the past 100 years has been based on averages from groups. This is called a nomothetic approach. But, as you may know, someone six feet tall can drown in a lake with an average depth of four feet.

Fortunately, we are at the beginning of the age of idiographic science, that is, a science focused on individuals (Fisher, 2015; Fisher et al., 2018). New ways of doing idiographic research and new forms of statistical analysis are being developed, as well. Many counselors and psychotherapists are also realizing that a focus on "disorders" has its limitations. Practitioners are becoming more interested in helping their clients do better overall. "Curing" the "disorder" is not their primary concern.

In 2005, Norcrass and Goldfried noted that

> much of the opposition to eclecticism should properly be redirected to *syncretism* [italics in original]—uncritical and unsystematic combinations (Norcross, 1990; Patterson, 1990). This haphazard "eclecticism" is primarily an outgrowth of pet techniques and inadequate training, an arbitrary, if not capricious, blend of methods by default. . . . Eysenck (1970, p. 145) characterized this indiscriminate smorgasbord as a "mish-mash of theories, a hugger-mugger of procedures, a gallimaufry of therapies," having no proper rationale or empirical verification. This muddle of idiosyncratic and ineffable clinical creations is the antithesis of effective and efficient psychotherapy. (pp. 15–16)

It is now almost 20 years later, we have even more schools and techniques than we had in 2005 and many more than in 1990, and therapists and counselors often call their approach "eclectic." In response, this book advocates for a combination of, at its core, evidence-based approaches, with the addition of other healing strategies. It does not advocate for "uncritical and unsystematic" combinations or a "hugger-mugger of procedures." In contrast, it advocates for a reasoned, structured approach that may include non-evidenced techniques that have worked for a client. It is up to scientists to investigate and understand why they may have worked rather than dismiss them as foolish rituals or the result of the placebo effect. It is time to open our scientific inquiries into realms that are inexplicable and mysterious to us.

INTEGRATING APPROACHES FROM OTHER CULTURES

CBT researchers and practitioners were the first to fully embrace evidence-based practice. It is called the "gold standard of treatment" (David et al., 2018). However, psychology is a very young science. Other ways of healing and improving the quality of life and relationships are just beginning to be investigated and what makes sense in one culture may not make sense in another. Over the past two decades, research has also shown that CBT is good, but other approaches are effective, as well. Moreover, research also indicates that 30%–50% of people do not respond to talk therapy or medication. What can be found to help them? An approach that integrates evidence-based approaches with approaches from other traditions and cultures may be the answer. Over the next hundred years, we will learn a great deal more about other approaches to healing in other cultures and other parts of the world and how they work. It will be an exciting time for those who are curious and love to learn.

SESSION STRUCTURE

From my own experience in psychoanalytic therapy and my readings of the works of Carl Rogers, Rollo May, Fritz Perls, and others, I realized that most counselors and therapists did not follow a structure in their sessions. However, the more I worked, especially with people who had limited budgets and time, I saw that my clients would benefit if I had a structure in mind. No good counselor or therapist would follow it blindly or in a manualized manner. But they wouldn't only listen and occasionally speak in a session either. Good, modern counseling and therapy sessions usually have a structure, including the following six parts:

1. building the working alliance and enhancing hope and motivation,
2. ongoing assessment, including assessing between-session experiences,
3. discussing and agreeing on therapeutic goals,
4. setting the agenda,
5. in-session work, and
6. agreeing on between-session work.

Of course, how closely you follow the structure will depend on the client and what they are bringing into the session. The first part of this book's organization follows this structure. Each of the first six chapters suggests what you could do in each part of a session. Given that each client is different, what you and your client choose to do will vary.

FOUR MAIN THEORIES

Psychology is too young a science to have a unifying theory. Even physics, a much older science, does not have one. However, four fundamental overlapping theories can guide us in our efforts to provide the best care possible:

The Stages of Change, Transtheoretical Model (TTM)

When I started, the stages of change model was quite new. Prochaska and DiClemente had published their seminal article in 1982 (Prochaska & DiClemente, 1982; Prochaska, DiClemente & Norcross, 1992). It proposed that everyone goes through stages of change no matter what behavior they are trying to change, from how they talk to their child, how they hit a golf ball, how they cut down on drinking alcohol or smoking cigarettes, or how they manage their moods and emotional responses. There have been a number of legitimate criticisms of the model (Bunton et al., 2000; West, 2005), but clinicians and clients love it, and many studies support its effectiveness (e.g., Krebs et al., 2018). Clinicians and clients can easily understand the model, and it helps them understand and accept the frustrating nature of change. Change often occurs in fits and starts, with two steps forward and one step back being quite common. Starting out, this model was a great help to me. It helped me decide what technique or approach to use with whom and when. Techniques that worked well with someone in a later stage of change would not help with someone in an early stage.

According to the model, initially a person doesn't think about changing. They're in Stage I, Pre-contemplation. Then they start to think about it, but they're not sure. They're ambivalent about changing. They're in Stage II, Contemplation. During Stage III, Preparation, they start to investigate and consider ways they might change. Maybe they check up on something online or they buy new sneakers for going to the gym. In Stage IV, Action, they start to try to change. Commonly, in the beginning, they're not very successful. They slip back to contemplating, thinking, for example, *Is this really worth it? Do I really need to change?* In Stage V, Maintenance, they've changed their behavior and that change is fairly stable. Their goal now is to maintain the change. For example, they've lost weight or stopped smoking cigarettes. Now they have to focus on keeping the weight off or not smoking again. In Stage VI, Termination, they're done. They've changed, and they don't have to pay much, if any, attention to the problem behavior.

However, some psychological difficulties may never go away. It is better for clients to remain in Maintenance mode. They can always easily gain weight again and, given the right combination of factors, panic attacks may return. For many people who have addictive problems, such as with alcohol, it may be dangerous to ever think *I've got it. I don't have to worry about this anymore.* In fact, that kind of thinking almost always leads to a relapse. The same is true for depression. If people stop doing what is keeping them healthy, for example, exercise, meditation, and therapy, they will be more prone to becoming depressed again.

A major positive aspect of the model is that it asserts that going back and forth between stages is common. That helps clients work on remaining hopeful, determined to change instead of feeling frustrated, angry, and full of shame when they slide backward. Almost everybody succeeds and fails and fails and succeeds as they work on changing. They are not defective, weak, awful people. They can work on accepting that that is the norm. Thankfully, positive change is the norm, despite what many people believe (Bishop, 2018; Calabria et al., 2010; Esser et al., 2014; Lopez-Quintero et al., 2011).

Some people leapfrog over the stages (Miller, 2004; West, 2005). They quite suddenly change. Were they quietly thinking about it and preparing? Such sudden change, what Dr. William Miller, the creator of motivational interviewing, calls "quantum change," is not well researched or understood. But such sudden change means that the theory does not fit everyone all the time. The theory has also been criticized for ignoring the impact of factors outside the individual, such as racism, cultural norms, etc. (Bunton et al, 2000). But the model does not attempt to explain the causes of change. It simply outlines what is common in the way people change.

The Cognitive Behavioral Model

Obtaining my PhD was delayed by family responsibilities, but without a PhD, I could not obtain a license in New York State to be a psychologist. Before getting my degree, I went for therapy for three years. My therapist was a psychologist-in-training who was primarily influenced by object relations, psychoanalytic theory. It was very helpful in many ways. But it was also very slow.

I knew I needed a lot of training before I started to work as a therapist, and I needed a supervisor. I had read about an interesting new form of therapy, cognitive therapy. However, Beck's training institute was in Philadelphia, and my family obligations prevented me from going there. I had heard about the Institute for Rational Emotive Therapy run by Ellis, so I went to one of his Friday night demonstrations. For $5.00 you could watch two volunteers working with him, and there was a coffee and donuts social hour afterward. Ellis wanted to "give psychology away," and this was his way of doing it.

I'm not sure that Ellis was a fan of the comedian Lenny Bruce (seen in the TV series *The Marvelous Mrs. Maisel*) who was famous for using the f-word throughout his gigs, but Ellis's demonstrations were similar. Jokes and four-letter words flew through the packed room. I didn't like what I saw. But his institute was the only one in New York offering training in a form of CBT he called, at that time, rational emotive therapy (RET). I signed up for the week-long workshop. Fortunately, Ellis behaved quite differently in his office with the moderately small group of 22 trainees. The first three hours were the best I had spent in the past 10 years. He was clearly part philosopher and part psychologist. He demonstrated an amazing memory and intelligence, and he clearly encouraged an integrative, not just RET, approach, which I liked very much, even at that time.

Ellis is the grandfather of CBT. He started with rational therapy (RT) in 1955 but quickly realized that emotions were key to human functioning and to counseling and psychotherapy. RT became RET, rational emotive therapy, and then finally REBT, rational emotive behavior therapy in 1993. CBT asserts that emotions, thinking, and behavior all interact and affect each other. It is based on a much older philosophy, Stoicism. Epictetus, the founder of Stoicism, believed that nothing that happened to you caused the way you feel. It is what you think about what has happened or is happening that is the real cause. If you want to change the way you feel or are behaving, change your thinking. Acceptance was key to Stoicism. That was primarily because Epictetus believed in God and whatever happened was the will of God. It was pointless to upset yourself about it. That would just make things worse.

Many people adopted Stoicism as an excellent guide to how to live a happier, fuller life, including the Roman emperor, Marcus Aurelius. However, according to Bertrand Russell, Stoicism lost out to Christianity because life became too difficult near the end of the Roman empire. People needed something to give them hope and help them get through such dreadful times. Christianity offered hope and the idea that something better was possible (i.e., life after death and heaven).

CBT should probably be called CEBT, cognitive emotive behavior therapy. I once asked Ellis why he didn't call his therapy cognitive emotive behavior therapy. "Because nobody knew the word back then," he said. "It existed, but it wasn't until Neisser wrote his book (in 1970), *Cognitive Psychology* that it became popular."

It is easier to work directly on our thinking and our behavior than to work on our feelings, so most practitioners also focus more on a client's cognitions and behaviors, and it is easy to neglect the emotive piece. Fortunately, Dr. Les Greenberg and others have helped fill the gap with emotion focused therapy (EFT; Greenberg, 2011).

By itself, CBT has helped many people, but every therapist also knows that it does not resonate with or help all clients.

The Neurochemical Theory, Medical Model

Prozac entered the market in 1985, and the creation of hundreds of other psychotropic medications revolutionized the field. The neurochemical theory is not as strong and foolproof as the pharmaceutical companies and most psychiatrists would like to have us think, but it can be extremely important for effective modern therapy with some clients.

Changing our neurochemistry changes how we feel, think, and behave. But we now know that medications are not the only way to affect such changes. Talk therapy, exercise, and medication are just three well-researched ways (see chapter 19 for many others). Nevertheless, some clients will definitely benefit from medications, even though we are not sure how they work.

Helping people accept the way their unique neurochemistry changes as the result of daily, monthly, and seasonal rhythms is also key to helping them think, feel, and do better. Unfortunately, we do not yet know how to predict the impact that a confluence of such rhythms may have on psychological distress, resulting in panic attacks, depression, bipolar disorders, addictive behaviors, etc., but we are learning more each year.

The PRIME Theory

In 2012, still trying to better understand how people change, I came upon Dr Robert West's PRIME model (West & Brown, 2013). Although it is still not well known, West, formerly professor of health psychology at the University College in London, proposes that a number of factors must come together before psychological problems appear, such as depression, panic attacks, or relapse to some form of addictive behavior. Humans tend to look for one factor when they are trying to figure out what is wrong. This is true whether they are trying to figure out why their car won't start or why they feel so miserable. In the past (and this is still true for some clients today), if they were troubled, they thought, *I didn't make enough offerings to the gods.* Nowadays many clients think: *It's because of my trauma* or *Maybe I need some form of medication.* However, it is more probable that several factors have come together to cause a problem. Specifically, West argues that seven factors, affected by feedback loops and feed-forward loops, interact to cause a client's behavior:

1. External factors, activating events: Relationship problems, unsupportive peers, employment problems, cultural factors, systemic racism, religions, political upheavals.
2. Internal factors: Genetic predispositions, neurochemistry, drives, reactance levels, and ideas about identity(ties), beliefs, values.
3. Conditioning/habits—some functional/helpful and some not.
4. Responses: The emotional, behavioral, cognitive responses to the internal and external factors.
5. Evaluations: The above responses are always being evaluated in terms of underlying beliefs, values, goals (7) and plans (8).

6. Feedback loops: Responses (4) and evaluations (5) interact and affect each other. For example, in response to being yelled at by their boss (1), their reactive nervous system and various beliefs (2) (*I can't stand being yelled at*) contribute to their leaving the office (4) which they evaluate (5) (*I'm such an ass. I ran away, like I always do*). That starts a feedback loop: run away, think ill of self, go home, watch hours of TV, think more ill of self, go to sleep very late, don't go to work the next day. . . .
7. Goals: Besides keeping safe and feeling less vulnerable, your client's goals may include a desire to develop a more meaningful job and/or a different self or identity.
8. Plans: In order to achieve those goals, a client needs plans and needs to check, with your help, whether or not they are working.

It is a complex theory, but I think most readers would agree that life is complex and most humans that we meet are even more complex than we ever imagined, including ourselves.

PRIME theory suggests that if one factor is changed everything else will change. That means that if your client changes one factor—their thinking, perhaps as a result of therapy with you, or a behavior, for example, drinking less coffee or resuming meditation—the way they feel, think, and behave will change.

OTHER THEORIES

Some readers may wonder why I didn't include attachment theory (Bowlby, 1979; Vicedo, 2020), trauma theory (Brown, 2004; Frankel, 1998) and/or polyvagal theory (Porges, 2011). I also could have included one or more of the many neo-Freudian theories created by Jung, Adler, Klein, Kohut, Sullivan, Erickson, and Horney. As noted earlier, there are literally hundreds of "schools" with their distinct theories, all attempting to explain human behavior.

Freud's theories are not supported by scientific evidence, but they still have a profound effect. Many clients and therapists continue to believe that the subconscious is largely made up of socially unacceptable sexual and aggressive thoughts and feelings. Dr. James Jackson Putnam, Harvard professor, the first president of the American Psychoanalytical Association, and the man perhaps most responsible for promulgating Freud's ideas in the United States, tried valiantly to persuade Freud that most humans have more positive impulses and were capable of doing wonderful things, but Freud was unmoved (see *Putnam Camp* [Prochnik, 2012] by Putnam's grandson, a wonderful book about, among other things, the trip made by Freud, Jung, and Firenzi to Putnam Camp in the Adirondacks in 1909).

The results of the adverse childhood events (ACE) study (Felitti et al., 1998) suggest that Freud's original seduction theory was probably correct (Esterson, 1998; Gay, 1998; Masson, 2012, McCullough, 2001). Some or many of the "hysterical" patients he was treating were being abused by male family members. Freud's revised theory, that the women were fantasizing, caused the field to look inward for repressed and highly defended against ideas rather than focus on outside factors, such as real abuse and trauma. Clinicians started to look for the causes in the women, blaming the victim, in many cases. Unfortunately, considerable harm may have been done by many well-meaning clinicians.

About 10 years ago, I was reading about monastic life in medieval Europe. I came upon the following passage written by a monk:

Textbox 2.1. Case—Sarah: Six Factors Combine for a Perfect Storm

Sarah, a wonderful, funny, hard-working young woman, had had a panic attack after months of not having one. Together, we looked for the factors that might have come together to trigger it. It turned out that Sarah had gradually begun to drink more coffee. That was because she was not sleeping as well as she had been and was feeling tired during the day. She had recently been given a promotion, which she was very happy about, but she had new, added responsibilities. She had to do some quick learning and was anxious that she might not be up to the task. Worrying kept her awake: *If I lose this job, I'll never get another one. I'll feel so ashamed. How will I ever be able to face my friends?* Her job now took more time, so she had been skipping meditation classes and not going to the gym.

We hypothesized that six factors had come together to cause the panic attack: (1) A new job with more work. (2) She had always been ambitious to do well in her job, and thoughts about possibility failing—*I must not fail. I absolutely could not stand getting fired! What would I do?*—created a feedback loop: more worrying, less sleep; less sleep, more worrying. (3) That led to often feeling tired. She hated feeling tired. To her, *Only lazy people feel tired.* (4) So, she upped her caffeine intake, creating another feedback loop: more caffeine, poorer sleep, more fatigue, more caffeine, poorer sleep, more fatigue. (5) She had stopped meditating. (6) She didn't think she had time for exercise and didn't feel like doing it.

Six factors came together to upend Sarah's hope of never having a panic attack again. I hypothesized that her thoughts that she had to succeed and absolutely could not stand being fired were the result of childhood trauma. I knew that if we could help her process that trauma, it would help her going forward. But I also knew that that might take a long time. Perhaps we could reduce the likelihood of another panic attack if we could alter one of the other contributing factors in the coming week. In her case, she chose two factors to change: her caffeine intake and a return to her meditation practice, which she said had been very helpful in the past.

Between sessions, she decided to try to pour herself half a cup every time she went to get coffee, and she tried to increase the time between cups. She also decided to not drink any caffeine after 4:00 p.m. In session, we worked on processing where and when she may have developed the beliefs: *I must not fail in this job. It would be terribly humiliating if I did.* We worked to help her develop new, kinder beliefs that would not only help her enjoy life more but, at the same time, eliminate other factors that might contribute to another panic attack.

The following session, in checking on how things were going, she told me that she had reduced her caffeine intake, was sleeping better, was less tired during the day, and had started meditating again. She had had no new panic attacks. Of course, not all clients are so successful at changing one or more of their behaviors between sessions, but many can and do. As a result, they can function better while they are working on other issues in therapy, for example, trauma.

In church, the devils make us sing badly. One day, when the Abbot's choir was beginning the first psalm for Matins, the devils came crowding in and, by going to and fro, made the brothers quickly break down in the singing. When the other side of the choir tried to put them right, the devils, flying across, so disturbed them that they no longer knew what they were singing. The Prior saw a devil like a white-hot iron come out of the mouth of one monk . . . and fly across to the other side. And he knew the cause of all the mischief.

I don't believe in "little devils," but what impresses me is how convinced the writer and the prior were of the correctness of their theory. For centuries people also believed that the sun went around the earth and that we were the center of the universe. It was so clear and apparent! In fact, you can still collect evidence and "prove" it to yourself every uncloudy day. The sun comes up in the east and sets in the west, going around the earth. It's obvious. The takeaway? Even if the evidence seems very apparent, the reality may be very different and the theory very wrong. At this point in time, it is important to remain open to new theories but also skeptical.

METASTABILITY AND BEHAVIORAL "STORMS"

In 2015, I started reading about apps that could help predict when a person suffering from a bipolar condition was becoming depressed or manic. Many bipolar people are not aware that they are getting depressed or manic until their condition has become very severe. Theoretically, the app could warn them. At the time, I was also working with clients who overdrank. Some met the criteria for "alcohol abuse," then the term used in the *DSM-III*, but some did not. However, they often drank much too much, leading to problems at work and in their personal relationships. They were also usually surprised that they had gotten so drunk. I wondered if we could predict overdrinking like we predict the weather. That led me to buy a book, *Forecast*, by Mark Buchanan. In it he discussed a concept new to me, "metastability" (Kelso, 2012; Kringelbach & Berridge, 2017). Here was a new way of thinking about sudden, negative changes that cause so much distress for people, not just those who overdrink but those who have panic attacks or who suddenly lose their temper (one could say they have "anger management attacks").

It turns out that appearing stable but not actually being stable is quite common in nature. This phenomenon is called metastability. The best example of metastability is a mountain before an avalanche. Everything looks stable, and then something, perhaps quite small, triggers a huge change in "behavior." Then everything looks stable again. But is it really?

Neural modular networks help manage our behavior. One network helps us drive the car as the other manages the conversation that we are having with our friend. If a truck suddenly lurches out from a side street, the driving network will quickly take over and, hopefully, save our lives. If our conversing network were very stable, the driving network might not be able to take over fast enough, and we might die. The lack of stability—the inherent metastability of your brain—saves the day. However, for many of our clients, this lack of stability creates problems. At 7:00 p.m., they are doing fine. But at 8:00 p.m. they are feeling depressed and eating the entire pint of Häagen-Dazs ice cream.

People and weather systems are similarly complex. Storms "behave" in certain ways given a number of internal and external factors. For example, it takes four factors to cause a tornado. Meteorologists use the acronym SLIM to remember the four factors: shear, lift, instability, and moisture. One day, the weather may look very ominous but nothing terrible happens. The four factors must be present and to the right degree to spawn a tornado. Something similar may take place when people relapse to depression, panic attacks, overdrinking, etc. Various factors come together and then what looks perhaps to both you and your client as reasonably stable suddenly changes.

THE ROLE OF TIME AND FEEDBACK LOOPS

Feedback loops also made Sarah's problems worse. We don't talk much about the significant impact of feedback loops in counseling and psychotherapy, although Ellis and others have written about "secondary problems" (Ellis, 2003). A "positive feedback loop" increases whatever is changing. In the case of a fire, more heat leads to more flames, which leads to more heat, which leads to more flames. In Sarah's case, less sleep led to the consumption of more caffeine, which led to even less sleep.

Many people who have a variety of psychological difficulties can make matters worse through feedback loops. For example, a client may wake up and feel depressed. A slight feeling of depression in the morning does not necessarily presage the coming of a full bout of depression, but they may think, *OMG, I'm getting depressed again* and stay in bed. Then they may lie in bed thinking about how awful their last bout of depression had been and of all the bad things that had happened. Normally, they would have thought about how a nice hot cup of tea or coffee would taste, and they would have gotten up and started the day. But the depression about the depression keeps them in bed. This feedback-loop-induced problem is such a critically important factor that Ellis argued that it was more important to address the depression about the depression first.

Clients can bring on full-fledged panic attacks via positive feedback loops. If they feel even a tiny twinge of anxiety, perhaps triggered by something completely outside of their consciousness, they think, *OMG, I might be getting a panic attack. I can't stand it if that happens. I would look so stupid.* Those thoughts may lead to tightening in their body. Your client *is* stuck inside the body of a mammal. Should they fight or run or freeze? The tightening in the body, specifically the chest, may lead to a small oxygen/carbon dioxide imbalance that the brain senses. In response, it sends adrenalin into the system, leading to more twinges, more awfulizing and catastrophic thinking, and eventually to a full-blown panic attack.

MANAGING "THE COMMITTEE": NEURAL MODULAR NETWORKS

"Neural modular networks" is a mouthful, so I prefer to refer to them as "the Committee."

Most people, perhaps all, have conflicting voices in their heads, not psychotic voices, but voices arguing for one action over another during the day: *Work another half hour. Take a break. No, don't take a break. Send that email. No, work on it some more.* Some neural networks may have been created when your clients were young. As a result, a "committee member" may toss up the idea that they can't do what they had set out to do: *You'll probably get it wrong* or suggest, *Check Instagram first.* Fortunately, more mature, goal-focused committee members may object to such ideas, and your client will get down to work. Learning to manage such committee member ideas is key to doing better and will be discussed in greater length throughout the book.

PART II

Initial In-Session and Between-Session Work: Step-by-Step

Chapter 3

Step 1: Build the Working Relationship: Enhance Hope and Motivation

All healers work to build hope and expectations in their clients or patients. Psychiatrists, psychoanalytically trained therapists, and most healers in other cultures tend to rely on a top-down model. They are the experts. They know. They signal their power in a number of ways. They put up diplomas on the wall, wear a lab coat or large gold necklaces. Many work in special buildings, designed to impress. They may be referred to as Dr. so-and-so while the client's first name is used. The goals are twofold: Establish who the expert is and raise hope and expectations.

In contrast, an existential therapist may appear in sandals, insist on relating on a first-name basis, and indicate in many other ways that the client and they will work in a collaborative manner. They are equals. All of this signals a very different kind of relationship, but the fact that it breaks the rules may also be designed—consciously or unconsciously—to raise hope and expectations: This is different. It will work.

Obviously, all of these signaling devices can and are manipulated whether you want to acknowledge it or not. The fact that you wear sandals, a lab coat, or a gold necklace is not an accident. But the message is always the same: I can help. Ellis had T-shirts and mugs and pencils to sell in his institute in New York City. He consistently used four-letter words in his demonstrations. They all helped to increase hope: This is different. It will work!

I know a wonderful therapist who works in New York City with teenagers with problems. He studies Buddhism, so you might expect him in sandals. But he is always dressed in a suit and a tie and formal, polished, tie-up shoes. The message is clear: This is business. I am a professional. On the other hand, he is very relaxed with a great sense of humor and uses humor extensively in his sessions.

The client in your office may have already read about a particular form of therapy online, as the newest, scientifically proven, and best therapy available. What are they looking for? Probably a talk therapy that is different. If you follow the suggestions in this book, your session will, in fact, look and sound quite different from standard, traditional therapy. Besides wanting to know the client's goals, you may teach something useful in the very first session, and you may suggest some kind of work that the client can do between sessions. You will probably do 30% to 50% (hopefully, not more) of the talking in the session, so the session will be more like a conversation. If the session goes well, your client will leave with their hopes increased, feeling that they have been heard and understood—to a point that is reasonable given the lack of time—and with something or several practical things to do as "homework." You have worked this way intentionally to raise your client's hopes and expectations.

Most clients are ambivalent about changing. Given the expense and time involved, it is no wonder that so many people are ambivalent about even starting therapy, especially if they come from a poor community where financial means are limited, and they are working two jobs or from a culture that still sees therapy and counseling as only for the mentally "sick." And change almost always involves discomfort. Who is not ambivalent about experiencing discomfort even if the long-term goal is desired?

Moreover, clients' motivation—often much to their dismay—varies by the day and hour. This is much clearer if you work with people who are trying to moderate or stop some form of addictive behavior, but it is true for almost all clients, as well. One member of a couple may be quite ambivalent about coming to therapy. A depressed person may not want to expend the energy to get up and come to your office. Many "anger management" clients do not want to give up their angry outbursts.

Hope and an expectation that things will get better increases a person's motivation. When I sat down in my first session running a group with Ellis, he looked at the person sitting next to him and asked, "Okay. What do you want to work on?" I learned later that that was Ellis's classic first line, and it was always said with great emphasis and assurance. Its tone was full of hope and expectation. Something positive was about to happen. It was motivating. "Let's get down to work and get a handle on this problem," it seemed to say.

Dr. Marsha Linehan, the founder of dialectical behavioral therapy (DBT), often uses a strong and sometimes irreverent style for a similar reason. Dr. Steve Hayes, the creator of acceptance and commitment therapy (ACT), and its practitioners are very explicit about the motivating power of values, acceptance, and commitment. "What are you willing to do?" they ask. There are two whole chapters on "willingness" in the book *Get Out of Your Mind & Into Your Life* (Hayes & Smith, 2005). The title and the book with its many exercise sheets and its focus on acceptance and commitment raise expectations and increase hope and motivation to change.

Research suggests (Cuijpers et al., 2019; Flückiger et al., 2018; Norcross & Lambert, 2018; Norwood et al., 2018) that the quality of the working relationship may contribute more to the effectiveness of counseling and psychotherapy than any other factor. Moreover, low or no empathy may not only make for ineffective therapy but may also be harmful. In their research, Moyers and Miller (2013) found that "High-empathy counselors appear to have higher success rates regardless of theoretical orientation. Low-empathy and confrontational counseling, in contrast, has been associated with higher dropout and relapse rates, weaker therapeutic alliance and less client change" (p. 878).

WHAT CAN YOU DO?

Take Notes During the Session

I know that many counselors and psychotherapists are still trained to write their case notes after a session. This is based on the idea that you can't take notes and listen carefully at the same time, although I don't think there is any research to support that notion. Freud took notes during the session. Most medical doctors do so now, as well.

In addition, something may happen right after the session. Your boss or spouse may call. Then you have to wait until the end of the day or after dinner to write your case notes. At that point, you will not remember as well as you would like and that may make you start to feel guilty and to start hating your profession. Next step? Burnout. It's important to make your work as enjoyable as possible and to be able to leave your work at the office. Self-care and how

Textbox 3.1. Research Note #2: What You Think About a Client May Affect the Outcome

Many years ago, two researchers, George Leake and Albert King (Leake & King, 1977), studied the impact of counselor expectations on outcome, with some very surprising results. They showed that if a counselor thought more highly of some clients compared to others, the more highly regarded clients did better. Leake and King told the counselors in three different centers that certain individuals had scored higher on a "specially designed psychological personality test for hard-core alcoholics." The "special" test was a real personality test, but what the counselors were told was made up. The high scores, the counselors were told, indicated that those individuals had "'high alcohol recovery potential,' had high motivation to accept counseling and could be expected to show exceptional recovery from the counseling they were about to receive" (p. 17). The number of people in the study was small, 12, 17, and 22 in three separate centers, and the number of "high alcohol recovery persons" (HARPS) clients was even smaller, 3, 4, and 5. But I have never forgotten the results.

At the end of the year's program, not only did the counselors rate HARPS more highly, but so did the other participants in the program. How did that happen? At the start, all of the recovering individuals, both HARPS and non-HARPS, were very similar. They had all lost their jobs because of their drinking, all were unemployed, all had previous police records, and all had gone to AA. The participants were even similar on the personality test.

In evaluating everyone at the end of the program, counselors gave significantly higher ratings to the HARPS. They were rated as more motivated, more punctual, neater in appearance, demonstrating more self-control, and exerting more effort to stay sober.

The HARPS were frequently the first to be told about job opportunities that came in, presumably because the counselors thought they had a better chance of taking advantage of such an opportunity. And, in fact, they got and held on to more jobs than the non-HARPS.

But the HARPS were no different from the non-HARPS.

What the counselors thought about them seems to be the factor that made the difference.

So if you don't like someone or you don't think they'll do well, should you continue to see them or should you refer them out?

This study suggests that you should refer them out. Somehow, probably nonverbal behaviors that you can't or that are very difficult to control will signal to the client how you feel and think and that will make therapy less effective, maybe even ineffective or harmful.

---

you use your leisure time is critically important. Writing notes *during* the sessions is a major part of self-care. At the end of the session, you should be done. You can talk to a colleague, call someone, or go home.

Moreover, during the session, you can capture exactly how a client expressed themselves. A month later, remembering exactly how someone said something may be very helpful.

Make a Strange Relationship Less Strange

"How's Bella?"

Bella is my client's King Charles spaniel, and the most important "person" in her life. Bella was sick when my client, Clara, was previously in my office, and she was very anxious about her.

By starting with "How's Bella?" I am clearly signaling three things that I think are key to any good relationship: First, I *was* listening the last time we met. Second, I picked up on the fact that Bella is incredibly important to Clara. Third, I remembered. (Actually, I would not have remembered had I not put something in my notes about Bella and had I not reread my notes before Clara walked in. I don't have a good memory. Taking notes during the session and reading them before another session helps me overcome that problem.)

Is asking about Bella manipulative? No, I don't think so, any more than my saying hello and remembering to ask a friend about something significant in their life. It is critically important to start to build a trusting relationship from the very beginning. I don't want to be friends with my clients. But I do want to have a good working relationship, so remembering and asking about important things in their life is simply the sensible thing to do.

Ours is a strange relationship. We get paid to listen and talk to someone. We get paid to help them feel better. It helps to do what we can to normalize the relationship, but not too much. I routinely write in my notes things that I think may help build the relationship: the age, name, and gender of children, and where they are going to school; the name of a pet and something about him or her, etc. If the client is taking training lessons with their dog or if their cat is about to undergo an operation, I write that down. If a child is applying to colleges, I note that.

Then when the client returns, I open the session with, "By the way, before we start, is your cat okay?" or "Did your son finish his applications?" As Gregory Bateson (2000) once pointed out in a wonderful essay entitled "Why Do Frenchmen?" dogs sniff each other and ants touch antennae when they pass. Humans engage in "small talk." The tone and content of the answers we get help us quickly understand if the relationship is essentially unchanged. If the tone is a bit off, most people immediately begin to ask questions trying to find out what the cause of that change is. Is the person irritated? If so, what might be the cause? Are they stressed about something in their life? If so, it would probably be good to know that and to express sympathy.

After a few minutes of small talk, I usually ask about the problems that brought the person into my office. I also find out a bit more about their personal life. If a union worker is in my office, and I sense that they may think I'm just some kind of ivory-tower intellectual, I'll somehow work into the conversation that I've been a union member for more than 50 years, and that I started as a longshoreman. If I find out that someone has children and they're going to public school in New York City, I'll share that I raised five children in New York City and that they all went to public schools and did fine. If I find out that their children are going to private school, I leave that public school part out.

Is this type of disclosure okay? Yes. The approach advocated for in this book does not require that the therapist be a blank slate upon which patients can transfer their feelings about, perhaps, their mother or father. However, there are definitely things not to disclose, as is discussed at the end of this chapter.

Normalize the relationship but not to the point of becoming friends. Yours is a professional relationship and will work better if you keep it that way. You may be tempted or even asked to make it a more friendly relationship, but do not do so. If you and your client become friends and you work very hard together on the client's depression, relationship issues, or a semi- or full-blown addictive behavior, if they lapse or relapse, will they share that with you? They might not if you have become too friendly. They might think that it might injure the relationship. You might get annoyed or irritated. You might wonder why all of your hard work together is not paying off. Consequently, they may not share when things go wrong. This is especially true if the behavior in question is felt to be shameful.

Unless you work in a small town where it is unavoidable, never agree to go to someone's wedding or party. Once I overrode my rule and went to the art opening of a client, Svetlana. Her art looked fascinating based on the photos she had shown me. I really wanted to look at it on real canvases. I had not been at the exhibit more than 10 minutes when her father came over, dragging Svetlana's younger sister behind him and said in a very loud voice, "You have to work with Violet. You have helped Svetlana so much. I'm sure you can help Violet, too." Violet looked as if she were going to die right there on the spot. I may have looked the same. I excused myself as quickly as possible and left.

In a small town, you may be forced to be on a town committee or to socialize together, but the more you can keep your relationship a professional one, the better. Would you do therapy with a friend? I hope not. Many people go to a therapist for the very reason that they have problems they do not want to share with a friend.

It is sad that we cannot become friends with some of our wonderful clients. But we can't. An old client, Jake, called and suggested that we have coffee. He had always wanted us to have a friendly relationship, and we'd not seen each other for five years. For that reason, he thought it would not be unethical for us to see each other on a friendly basis. I agreed with that part of his reasoning, but I said, "I don't think this is in your best interest. What if something happens in your marriage or you become depressed again, then what? You won't have someone you trust—me—to turn to. I would love to get together for coffee, but it's not a good idea. You should save this relationship as a professional relationship just in case the gods make a mess of your life. I hope that that will never happen, but we never know."

He agreed. I have his folder on file just in case. But this is the most negative aspect of our profession. All other professionals can get together socially with a client. We shouldn't.

Goal for the First Session

The goal of the first session is to get a second session. The goal is not to convince a person to do long-term therapy, perhaps multiple sessions per week. But the goal is to get a second session. Many people who come to therapy, especially men, have thought about it for a long time. It would be truly unfortunate if they quit before that had hardly begun.

Use Motivational Interviewing

Clients who volunteer for demonstrations with famous therapists are usually highly motivated to change (or actors playing the role of clients). But many of our clients are not necessarily so. They have probably vacillated for months between calling and not calling a therapist. This may be especially true with a client from a different culture or clients grappling with identity issues (see chapter 17). If you have not taken a workshop on motivational interviewing (MI), that should probably be first on your list.

MI is currently being used around the world in doctors' and therapists' offices. At the time that the creator, Dr. William Miller, started to work with problem drinkers, counselors typically confronted clients in a harsh, shaming manner. According to that approach, it was critical to break down someone's "denial."

Miller, a researcher as well as a clinician, wondered whether those techniques were really warranted or as effective or as necessary as many people—who had often recovered with such treatment—said they were. He did a number of carefully designed studies, sometimes using videotaping, and found that confrontive approaches increased the likelihood that someone would relapse, not the reverse. Based on that research, he began to develop a kinder, more respectful approach that evolved into MI (Miller, 1995; Miller & Rollnick, 2012).

The major aspects of MI can be remembered using the acronym FRAMES:

F   Feedback regarding personal risks
R   Responsibility for change
A   Advice regarding change
M   Menu of change options
E   Empathy from the therapist
S   Support self-efficacy

The client is first asked to fill out a series of assessment instruments. Once they are processed, the counselor gives the client feedback based on the scores. For example, a young college student may be told that when his fellow classmates drink, they drink on average 3.4 drinks per "session." His average is 7.5. This information is provided in a nonjudgmental, factual manner. Then the counselor explains that the responsibility for change is in the client's hands. The "doctor" is not going to "cure" them or try to force them to change. Unlike traditional therapy, advice is then provided as to what type of changes could be made and how that might be done. A menu of change options is also offered. Throughout the session, the counselor expresses empathy for the client's position and attempts to be very supportive of self-efficacy.

A variety of strategies for motivating people to change are used in the first and subsequent sessions. The acronyms DEARS and OARS help practitioners remember how to work during a session. DEARS stands for:

D   Develop discrepancy (using a variety of in-session exercises, scaling questions, etc.)
E   Express empathy (using reflection and open-ended questions)
A   Amplify ambivalence
R   Roll with the resistance
S   Support self-efficacy (help/encourage the client to *give voice* to self-motivational
      statements)

Many people in therapy are ambivalent about doing what they may need to do to change. Highlighting the discrepancy between what they say they want to do and what they are doing—again, in a gentle, kind, and curious manner—often helps people decide to take some kind of action in the week ahead.

Many clients may also show signs of resistance. Historically, in the addiction field, resistance was met with confrontation. MI suggests rolling with the resistance instead, that is, not being confrontive but, instead, inquisitive, or perhaps changing the topic or the approach.

OARS stands for:

O   Open-ended questions
A   Affirmations (true statements about the client, what they have done well, their positive attributes—to build the working relationship and build hope)
R   Reflective listening; empathic responses
S   Summarizing

It is common to ask "yes/no questions," so-called closed-ended questions. For example, to a client who is depressed, "Did you take your medication? Did you manage to get out of the house?" Such questions often make people feel as if they're being interrogated and that the questioner is not really interested in their problem. Research suggests that asking "open-ended questions" works better: "How has your medication been working or not working for you?" and "How has getting out of the house been going for you?"

Active or reflective listening also helps a client to feel that you are curious and eager to learn what is happening in their life. With reflective listening, you "join" with a client and help the client feel validated. MI trainers stress the value and importance of reflecting more on affect than content. "It sounds like it makes you angry when you think about going on that trip" is better than "It sounds like you don't want to go on that trip." And then adding, "Why do you think that is?" will further help the client to feel that you are really interested and trying to understand.

MI also emphasizes the importance of eliciting change talk, using questions like:

1. What would you like to see change about your current situation?
2. What would changing *mean* for you?
3. What might happen if you didn't make any changes?
4. How do you think you might be keeping yourself stuck?
5. What could you and I do to help you become unstuck?
6. If you start to change, what would help keep you on track?
7. If you woke up tomorrow and the problem was gone, what would you do?

What MI practitioners like to call the "spirit" of the interview/assessment is key. Learning how to use open-ended questions and a nonjudgmental tone is critically important to doing a good MI-informed assessment.

Be Both Empathic and Helpful

Clearly, being empathic is extremely important in therapy. It helps clients feel better and builds the working alliance. Leaving your office with something to do in the week to come will also help; it will contribute to their feeling more hopeful and less helpless. They are not dependent on being in the office or online with you, their therapist, to feel better. That "something" may also provide new insight into a problem, which is the way traditional therapy works. But modern therapy is focused as much on the development of better skills as it is on insight.

Textbox 3.2. Case—Bea: Ups and Downs

I saw Bea for more than 23 years, on and off, as she became better and worse and better again as the result of a bipolar disorder. All humans are somewhat bipolar on a daily, monthly, or seasonal basis. No doubt, you know that you feel more positive and more energetic at certain times of the day than others. You may have also noticed that you have groups of days when you "do not feel good." You are not clinically depressed, but you do not "feel like yourself."

There were times when Bea and I thought we understood what triggered off a manicky period and/or a depressive period, but they also just seemed to happen without rhyme or reason. For Bea, it made planning and living and working very difficult, sometimes impossible.

When I first met her, I asked what her goals were in therapy. She answered in a clear, firm but aggravated voice: "Stay out of hospitals!" She had been hospitalized twice prior to my meeting her, and each experience had been, in her words, "a traumatic experience."

As do most people who have a true bipolar disorder, Bea resisted that label and what she perceived as the identity of being bipolar. For her, it meant that she was crazy, and, not surprisingly, she didn't want to be associated with such an identity. But she had other identities that she aspired to keep alive, although at times it was very, very difficult for her to do so. When she was doing better, she was a very friendly neighbor and kind aunt. When she was not doing well, she could be cantankerous and not at all pleasant to be with. Her biting, snarly remarks put people off, and she had lost a number of friends over the years.

One time during a seminar, someone asked Dr. Ellis whether he thought REBT could work with people who were psychotic, and he answered with one of his wisecrack remarks: "Better than anything else." But then he became serious, and noted that we, the people in the audience, could quickly tell that someone was psychotic or bipolar or had other serious mental health issues, and we moved away from them and avoided them. Consequently, they were left to make friends only with other people who were seriously disturbed. And those people frequently did not know how to be good friends. So often they were alone.

Bea was like that. If she made a friend, the friend often was a difficult person to interact with. One would sometimes get so angry with the other that they broke off the friendship. She was left with only family members and a few very old school friends.

Similar to almost every bipolar client I have worked with, initially, Bea could not accept that her neurochemical system behaved in such an erratic manner. How a therapist helps a client accept a serious diagnosis is probably more an art than a science.

Bipolar clients are, at times, manicky and cannot imagine that there is anything at all wrong with them. During such periods, they want to enjoy their period of "normality" and may not want to reflect on their problems. Helping a client accept that they do have a serious and difficult-to-handle health issue requires sensitivity, compassion, and honesty on the part of the therapist.

When depressed, Bea had so little energy that she could hardly get to my office. Her sleep was terribly distorted. She would fall asleep at 10:00 p.m. and then awaken at 1:00 or 2:00 a.m. and not be able to go back to sleep until 4:00 or 5:00 a.m., if at all. She would cancel medical appointments and miss get-togethers with friends, dates she had made with enthusiasm a week or so before.

She took six or seven different medications from an endocrinologist (for her diabetes), rheumatologist, cardiologist, and psychiatrist at different times during the day, and sometimes, perhaps because of some kind of diurnal or weekly or monthly rhythms that we do not yet understand, she would have a bad reaction to one.

When she was feeling better, she was also more feisty and had to be careful not to get in arguments—bordering on fights—with someone such as a friend or a pharmacist. She tried as best she could to practice preferential thinking: *They don't have to act the way I think they should act. I don't have to get it my way.*

At times, she wanted a homework assignment, but because she found it so difficult to do whatever she planned to do in the future, they often led to self-criticism and self-downing when she could not do them. Consequently, we had to be very careful about coming up with one and about talking about the "results" in the next session.

Talking about her childhood greatly helped Bea. Her mother had been hospitalized four or more times during her childhood. In contrast, her father had been very successful, and Bea had hoped to be like him. When that eluded her, it was helpful for her to remember that her mother had grappled with the same illness. I continually and consistently urged her to be gentle with herself, not self-critical and condemning. I encouraged her to realize that she was doing the best she could under the circumstances.

When she wanted to see me, I made time in my schedule to see her. She came in once a month or once a week, depending on how she was doing. Medicare and supplemental insurance made that possible. She was never hospitalized again. She died of a heart attack in her home at 72.

Do and Don't Disclose

I completely understand why psychoanalysts and some psychodynamic therapists do not share anything about their personal life with their patients (not "clients"; this model came out of the medical profession—Freud was a medical doctor, psychiatrist, and psychoanalyst). If I subscribed to a psychoanalytic theory, I would not share anything either.

According to the original psychoanalytic theory, repressed and strongly defended unconscious aggressive and sexual ideas—often repulsive to the patient and society—are the underlying cause of the problem. One of the key techniques, as you know, is (or was—it is not used very often now, at least in the United States) to have a patient lie on a couch looking away (very important) from the psychoanalyst, who sat behind and took notes. The objective was to have the client "transfer" thoughts and feelings onto the therapist, who acted as a kind of blank slate or screen. For example, the patient might transfer feelings of hate and aggression toward their mother, speaking seemingly at random (free associating). It was critically important that the psychoanalyst be a blank slate. Knowing anything personal about the therapist would destroy the effect. Because CBT and most of the other schools of psychotherapy listed in chapter 2 do not rely on transference, the therapist does not need to be a "blank slate."

For modern practitioners, Barnett (2011) provides a good guide regarding self-disclosure: Only disclose what happened to you and how you dealt with it IF: (1) it is in the rather distant past and (2) you have successfully worked it through. Otherwise, don't self-disclose.

For example, if I'm working with someone who is having a problem with procrastination, I may say, "I used to have a black belt in procrastination, but I don't anymore." I have shared that I had the problem, in fact, many years ago, and I have clearly signaled that the problem is solvable. That may help increase their motivation to continue to try to resolve the problem.

Ellis loved to tell stories from his own life. Whether they were true or not is irrelevant. He was trying to illustrate a point. Many people know how he said he overcame his fear of talking to women. According to him, he went to the Bronx Botanical Garden and spoke to an even 100, "good for research purposes," he used to say. Only one of them accepted his invitation for a date, and she didn't show up. But he was cured.

The story illustrates many key points: (1) One of the best ways to overcome a fear of something is to do it. (2) Few things are genuinely "awful" and generally you won't die. You'll just be very uncomfortable, which is a part of being human and striving to grow and change. (3) Often people take things much too seriously and make themselves miserable. The story is humorous for that reason. You can do it and stand the discomfort, especially if you don't make it so terribly important. And having a sense of humor about something will probably help you be less demanding about your performance, more accepting and less self-pitying.

In an extremely moving video (https://www.youtube.com/watch?v=tAz_o8G-67E), Linehan discloses the religious experience that changed her life and inspired her to develop DBT and to help other people who were in great distress, especially women. Hayes, in his TED Talk (youtube.com/watch?v=o79_gmO5ppg) shares in great detail how he overcame his panic attacks.

CAUTIONS

If you had or have a bad relationship with one or more parents, you may not want to share that even if you think the difficulties in the relationship have been resolved. Family relationships are extremely complex and difficult to understand. What you may think led to a better relationship may not have been the critical factor at all.

Do not share anything about your sexual life. That could easily be construed as being an attempt to talk about sex with a client with your own motives in mind. Your thinking about doing so may, in fact, be driven by a sexual attraction to the client, even if you are unaware of it at the time.

Chapter 4

Step 2: Initial Assessment

About a month into my training, during supervision, after I had described the difficulties I was having with a client, my supervisor said, "How would you conceptualize this in terms of an ABC?" I was stumped. Of course, I knew about the ABC model, but I had never thought about using it in my head to help me better understand a client's problems. As you will see by reading this chapter, there are many ways to assess a client's problems, and the approach that you use will probably be partly or totally determined by where you work, where you trained, and whether you are primarily a clinician or a researcher.

Assessment is an ongoing, session-to-session process. It starts in the first session, usually along with some work and perhaps an agreement to try doing something different between sessions. It continues in each session, often significantly helped by what occurs or does not occur between sessions. How you do assessment will also probably be determined by how much you have adopted motivational interviewing techniques, as discussed in the previous chapter.

Medical doctors are trained to evaluate a patient and then make a diagnosis: Lyme disease, COVID, IBS, and so on. In the past, psychoanalysts and psychodynamically trained therapists spent the first few sessions coming up with a diagnosis. The work did not begin until after the assessment and the diagnosis. In contrast, modern therapists usually combine assessment and some sort of work in the first session.

Assessing what is going on in the individual person sitting in front of you is complicated by several factors:

- Humans are one of the most complex phenomena in the universe. Black holes may be mysterious and little understood but in comparison to human individuals, they are less complex.
- Humans are complex primarily because they have a sense of time. They worry about what they have done in the past and what they may do (or not do) in the future. Without their ability to envision different, possible scenarios in the future, they would not make themselves anxious or depressed. Without envisioning scenes from the past, they would not cringe with discomfort, shame, humiliation, or feelings of depression. Without imagining being depressed in an hour, next week, and maybe forever, they would not make themselves more depressed. Humans and their place in time and their beliefs about their lives in time have a tremendous impact on their psychological problems.
- Humans are complex because they are interconnected and interdependent with everyone and everything around them. They are profoundly affected by these connections even though some people believe that they, themselves, are totally independent agents. But that belief, inculcated in some cultures more than others, can lead to serious problems in relationships, and to anxiety and depression, and addictive behaviors.

Most clinicians do not rely on their interviewing skills alone. They use some sort of assessment instrument prior to each session. Where you work may mandate that you do so. The Beck Depression Scale, the Beck Anxiety Scale, and the Beck Hopelessness Scale are three very popular ones, as is the PCL-5 for a traumatic experience. Some clinics use the Outcome Questionnaire 45 (OQ-45). The Veterans Administration's CBT program for substance use disorders uses their own assessment instruments. And the AUDIT is a very good, simple, free assessment instrument for alcohol use. Some clinics have clients answer questions on a tablet. Their therapist or counselor can see the results on their computer screen in their office before the client comes in.

In the first session, you may quite quickly have a variety of hypotheses as to what may be the causative factors involved. Based on those hypotheses, you will ask quite different questions. If you think the major reason for a problem is based in childhood trauma, you will probably spend quite a bit of the first session on learning about a client's childhood, perhaps without touching on the traumatic event or events because the client is not ready to do so. If you hypothesize that the problem may be based on overlearning/conditioning, you will try to understand what precedes and what follows a problematic event, for example, a bad argument with a partner or spouse or an episode of overdrinking.

Readers who are interested in one of the original forms of integrative assessment and therapy will find reading about Dr. Arnold Lazarus's work, multimodal therapy, very valuable (Lazarus, 1981). During my first six months at the institute, partly because he was a friend of Ellis's, I occasionally had the opportunity to chat with Lazarus in the waiting room. He created his own assessment approach, BASIC-ID. It was an acronym to help clinicians remember to explore the impact and interaction of a client's behaviors, affect, sensation (physical), imagery, cognition, interpersonal, and drugs. In studying it, I realized that the ABC/REBT/CBT approach that I was learning left out an assessment of sensations and imagery, and I started to assess clients in terms of all seven dimensions.

WHAT CAN YOU DO?

Don't Ignore or Undervalue Small Talk

As I noted in the previous chapter, the small talk when you greet someone in the waiting room or at the very beginning of a virtual session is a critical part of the first and ongoing assessments. "Small" is a very unfortunate term. Small talk is critically important. It helps us assess a relationship and, in our case, build a better one. What some people disparage as small talk is absolutely critical to maintaining good relationships with coworkers and family members. If a client can't be bothered with such "nonsense," they are like someone who wants a good garden but can't be bothered with weeding.

As you are engaging in small talk, you can observe the nonverbal language and what your client is wearing. You might be surprised how often clients who are depressed are dressed in grays, browns, and blacks, and as they start getting better, yellows, reds, and greens begin to appear.

Stages of Change Assessment

This form of assessment is designed to help you determine which stage of change your client is in and for which problem. You can use a formal stages of change assessment instrument (https:

//habitslab.umbc.edu/wp-content/uploads/sites/228/2014/07/University-of-Rhode-Island -Psychotherapy-Version-for-site.pdf) and/or you can use the model to better understand where your client is in terms of changing.

In your office, you will find the model helpful in two ways. Your client may be ambivalent about changing (Stage II, Contemplation), motivated and ready to change (Stage IV, Action), or only there because someone else made them come (Stage I, Pre-contemplation). Strategies that work with the first type of client will be a waste of time with the last type. They don't have a problem, at least, in their opinion.

Many of my clients who have been in my office with anger management issues are very ambivalent about changing their behavior. They like the short-term impact of their anger, even though it is ruining their personal relationships and may be interfering with their professional life. In contrast, people who are suffering from anxiety or depression or interpersonal problems are often very motivated. They want to feel less anxious or less depressed, and they want to find solutions to their relationship issues. Figuring out what stages they are in helps a clinician decide what to do next. This is especially true when they have multiple, interacting problems.

John, a very personable 45-year-old, was in my office because he was gaining weight, occasionally overdrinking, and reported being depressed and very anxious much of the time. He seemed eager to learn how to eat and drink in a more moderate fashion and also motivated to learn how to better manage his anxiety and depression.

Several times, I had noted during our talk that he made cutting, disparaging remarks about his wife and some of his coworkers, so I asked him, "What about anger? Is that something you would like to work on?"

"Why?" he said. "Do you think I have anger issues? No! That's not a problem for me."

He was in Stage I, Precontemplation, regarding his underlying anger. I noted that in my notes and in my mind and decided to work on something that he was more motivated to tackle and to return to that later.

CBT (ABC) Assessment

Ellis created the ABC(DE) technique or tool because he wanted clients to be able to do therapy on themselves between sessions. But the ABC model is also used for assessment by many CBT therapists. The ABC part of the ABC(DE) technique serves as an excellent way to gain insight into a client's beliefs and provides one way of assessing and conceptualizing a client's problems. Given an A (activating event), what are the client's beliefs (Bs) or automatic thoughts, which contribute to the Cs (consequences)? As an assessment technique, it is probably popular because it makes sense to a lot of clients.

CBT and Case Conceptualization

Dr. Aaron Beck (Beck, 1975), the creator of cognitive therapy (CT) in the 1970s, which has now evolved into CBT, was a medical doctor. He was looking for a cure for depression. "Case conceptualization" is a key part of the medical model. Dr. Windy Dryden, the author or editor of more than 200 books related to CBT, objects to the terms "case formulation" and "case conceptualization" because "the use of these terms perpetuates the objectification of clients. In short, a complex, unique person is objectified as 'a case'" (Dryden, 1998, p. 43).

Clients with their complex, interconnected problems can be overwhelming at times, especially for practitioners new to the profession. Hence, many clinicians find the kinds of methods and forms created by Dr. Christine Padesky and others (Liese & Esterline, 2015; Persons,

2012) to be extremely helpful. You may want to work collaboratively, hand in hand, with the client, even going as far as to suggest that the client help fill out the form with you in the office.

Padesky (2020) suggests several kinds of case conceptualization. One, in particular—Box/Arrow In/Arrow Out—is relatively easy to use. If you are working in person with a client, in the center of a piece of paper, draw a box about 2"x2", and then an arrow from the left pointing to the box and an arrow from the right leading away from the box. Ask your client what problem they would like to start with and write that in the middle of the box. Let's assume it is anxiety. Second, collect from the client the kind of situations or circumstances that trigger their anxiety and write those on the left side around the arrow pointing toward the box. Then find out how the client usually responds to anxiety and write those responses on the right side of the box. Then ask which of those responses make the anxiety better in the short run and to what extent they work over the long run. Finally, ask what other responses they can think of that might work better. Finally, you may want to ask what gets in the way of their using those strategies.

As you can see, one of the advantages of this assessment tool is that it easily shifts the focus to what might work better in the future. The assessment is not solely about the problem or what is contributing to the problem. It is also an assessment of what other strategies might be available to respond to the problem differently, specifically, in a more helpful manner. It is similar to Ellis's ABC model, but the client does not have to put beliefs in the box. Any problem can go in the box, making it a kind of functional analysis.

DSM-V, ICD-10 Assessment

In 1952, psychiatrists published the *Diagnostic and Statistical Manual* (*DSM*) which was modeled on the medical profession's identification of distinct, separate diseases. Unlike illnesses like malaria or COVID, it is difficult—some people would say impossible—to find the boundary between "normality" and a "disorder." The *DSM-V* has come under withering criticism by many people, including Dr. Allen Frances, the chair of the *DSM IV* Taskforce (Frances, 2013).

This book cannot teach you how to use the *DSM-5* or *ICD-10-CM*. However, assuming that it is critically important to you to function in an ethical manner, you also have an ethical responsibility to help your clients obtain the insurance reimbursement that they are entitled to. In cases where you don't feel as if a client is meeting the criteria for a more serious disorder, such as major depression or bipolar disorder, you may find that they meet the criteria for generalized anxiety disorder (GAD; 300.00 in the *DSM-5*; F41.1 in the *ICD-10-CM*) or you may opt for some form of adjustment disorder (309/F43). In many cases, you may not feel as if a client is exhibiting sufficient depression or anxiety to warrant 309.28, so you may opt for 309.9 (F43.20 in the *ICD-10-CM*), adjustment disorder, not otherwise specific (NOS). NOS is used in the medical field when it is not clear what is causing a problem. Given that some clients find some life events particularly difficult to adjust to, the diagnosis seems appropriate. However, to use it ethically and correctly, it is important to read the portion of the *DSM-5* and *ICD-10-CM* that applies to it.

PRIME Assessment

West's (West & Brown, 2013) PRIME model suggests a different way of looking at humans and their problems. The model's complex, interacting nature reflects the complex, interacting nature of human behavior and distress. As noted in chapter 2, the theory proposes that a number of factors must come together before a client feels or does something that is disturbing to them.

It is rare (and perhaps never occurs) that someone gets depressed or has a panic attack or relapses to an addictive or semi-addictive behavior because of only one factor or trigger or cause. It is not just because of trauma or an attachment problem as a child. It is not just because someone's neurochemistry became out of balance. Those factors very well may play a significant role, but no one factor will be sufficient. A number of factors must combine to create a problem (i.e., overwork or loss of a job, anger at a family member, lack of sleep, past familial trauma, and unhelpful core beliefs). Even if one factor may finally break the proverbial camel's back, other factors played a contributory role.

Working together, the client and therapist can try to identify which factors may be contributing to a problem and how they may interact. Then they can begin to figure out how best to resolve or manage the problem going forward.

FURTHER NOTES ON ASSESSMENT

Lumpers and Splitters, Transdiagnostic versus *DSM-5* and *ICD-10-CM/ICD-11*

Are you more of a "lumper" or a "splitter"? (Jaspers, 2003). Do you prefer to assess and diagnose in terms of the long list of disorders in the *DSM-5* and *ICD-11*? Or are you a lumper, preferring a transdiagnostic approach? Lumpers argue that mental illnesses are not like malaria and diabetes. The problems people can have in life should not be split up into 300-plus "disorders" (Dalgleish et al., 2020). People are in a therapist's office primarily because they are having difficulty in some important relationships, or they are not functioning well.

Splitters insist that it is vital to be able to specify and communicate effectively with other clinicians, including physicians, surgeons, physical therapists, and so on. This may be especially true if you are working in a large clinic or a hospital. The WHO's *ICD-11* has more than 55,000 codes for diseases, behavioral and mental disorders, injuries, and causes of death.

Behaving Ethically and Minimizing Harm

Unfortunately, the diagnoses that we file for insurance purposes do not always remain confidential. In one instance, the head of human resources at a large company in New York, overworked and extremely tired and stressed, had admitted herself into a hospital on a Thursday on my advice. She was unable to function and having suicidal thoughts. She was given some of the powerful medications now available and back at work on Tuesday. A month later, the EOB for her stay in the hospital happened to cross her desk. "Psychotic break" was the diagnosis. She quickly put it in the circular file (i.e., the trash basket).

Another executive was not so fortunate. He was diagnosed with social anxiety and alcohol misuse by a psychiatrist. There is no doubt that on occasion he overdrank, but whether or not he, in fact, met the *DSM-5*'s criteria for mild alcohol misuse or the *ICD-10*'s criteria is open to question. However, that is what the psychiatrist put down, and that information got out. He was not fired, but he didn't receive his expected promotion or any further promotions. This all occurred during a downturn in his industry, and he could not find another job. Incorrect diagnoses can harm people.

On the other hand, occasionally people who do meet the criteria for alcohol misuse or depression or bipolar disorder may want you to submit something not so serious, for example, generalized anxiety disorder, to their insurance company. Of course, you can't ethically do that.

Given their potential for promotions and future bonuses, you may want to suggest that they consider not submitting anything at all for insurance.

The world is as it is. No one can guarantee that once a number gets into a computer it will stay there forever or that the system won't get hacked. Consequently, it is very important to be careful about the diagnostic numbers that are provided for insurance purposes.

What Is Already in the Computer?

You may want to use the diagnosis and number a previous clinician has entered into the system if you agree with it. Of course, if you don't, you will enter what you think is the more correct number. However, if you are comfortable with the previous clinician's diagnosis and, ethically, you don't think you need to add another diagnosis, that may be the best route to take. If you are working in a hospital or clinic, it may want to you put down all of the diagnosis numbers that you think fit. In a medical setting, it may be critical for another practitioner to know that the patient has had triple bypass surgery, has diabetes, has AIDS, and is on high cholesterol medication. You may feel similarly about psychological disturbances. If so, all code numbers should be included in your notes.

The Cultural Formulation Interview

You may want to incorporate questions from the cultural formulation interview (CFI) to guide not only your initial and ongoing assessment but the way you work. If the CFI were more widely used, it would change the way clinicians in multicultural settings do assessments and view their clients. The emphasis is on how clients view their problem and not on how a clinician views their problems. How family, friends, and other members of their culture may be able to help is also integral to the CFI (Lewis-Fernández et al., 2020).

Clinicians versus Researchers

Researchers and clinicians who work in clinics, hospitals, or as solo practitioners have very different reasons for doing an assessment. Consequently, the way they assess clients differs significantly.

To obtain promotions and eventually a tenured position, researchers have to be very careful about which type of instruments they use and how well those instruments have been validated. They often decide to exclude people with multiple problems, the very type of people that clinicians encounter in their offices.

Personnel in a hospital and clinic have to assess in a similar manner and maintain careful records so that they can communicate effectively among themselves over time. However, for clinicians working alone in private practice, the way they assess will probably depend mostly on which theory or theories inform their work, which is usually a reflection of where they chose to get training. In fact, assessment instruments are often not used unless the clinician works at a university or private clinic.

Interpersonal Issues and Insurance

Marital counseling is not covered by most insurance plans. Other relationship issues, for example, between a client and their child, are also not covered. Given that the system we are working in is based on a medical model, unless there exists a codable "illness" or "disorder," insurance will not pay. Someone in the relationship is going to have to accept having a diagnostic number attached to their name.

Some people argue that all "mental illnesses" are the result of problems in relationships. They assert that even mood disorders and problems with emotional dysregulation have their roots in relationship problems and not in brain diseases, even though one's brain may become quite disordered or "diseased" as the result of long-term, ongoing neglect, abuse, or stress. As a result, someone in the relationship is probably really suffering from depression or anxiety or both. Consequently, you can give that person a diagnosis number, and they will probably get reimbursement from their insurance company.

Therapy and Sleuthing; The Columbo Technique

The Columbo technique is one of my favorite techniques when the client and I are a bit stuck. I learned it from Dr. Ray DiGiuseppe, the director of professional training at the Albert Ellis Institute, and one of my supervisors while I was a fellow there doing my postdoc. He and many others at the time were fans of the television series, *Columbo* (still viewable on YouTube and late-night TV). In *Columbo*, the actor Peter Falk plays a seemingly perennially confused detective in an old, shabby trench coat. At the beginning of each show, the viewer can tell that he has a long list of hypotheses regarding the possible suspects. He was best known for asking each suspect an annoying number of questions. When the suspect finally thought he was done, inevitably, Falk would turn around, scratch his forehead, and say, "I just have one more question." And, of course, that was the zinger.

What's the point? Therapy and sleuthing have things in common. We are trying to understand our clients, especially why they may be stuck in a certain kind of mood, behavior, relationship, or job. Because of shame or a lack of insight, they may not share some information that would be very helpful. At times, I find it very effective to look at someone in a quizzical manner, scratch my head, and say something like, "I'm confused. I thought you said you wanted to stop smoking pot, but you still go down in the basement and smoke a joint every night?" and I continue to look puzzled. Not judgmental but puzzled. The answer can be very helpful not only to me but for my client, too. They are often also confused and puzzled. Answering the question may motivate them to dig deeper.

When a client is sitting in front of you, I assume that you are trying to figure out what is going on.

If they are complaining about depression, it is probably due to a combination of factors. Which of the following do you think may contribute to their depression?

1. Past traumatic events in the client's life
2. Habits, including overlearned, conditioned avoidant responses
3. A disconnection with or displeasure of God or gods
4. A curse
5. Genetics
6. A neurochemical imbalance
7. Irrational/unhelpful beliefs, including cognitive distortions and core schemas
8. Pot, alcohol, or some other chemical, including medications
9. Not moving or exercising enough
10. Not sleeping enough
11. Job insecurity
12. Lack of meaningful, supportive personal relationships

13. Lack of purpose in life
14. Not accepting that it is in the nature of human life to suffer

Depending on how long you have worked, you may have a partial theory or hypothesis for what is going on after talking to a client for only a few minutes. Theories, conscious or unconscious, affect how we think about clients, how we assess, how we work, which of the above factors we think may be in play, and especially what questions we ask and when.

You can find a discussion of other ongoing assessment techniques, including homework as an assessment tool, in chapter 8.

Hidden Addictions?

Many clients who have addiction problems never bring them up with their therapists and many therapists never ask questions, especially about possible addictions to behaviors, such as shopping, watching porn, and video gaming. In her excellent book *Hidden Addiction*, Dr. Marilyn Freimuth (2009) discusses the fact that many therapists do not assess for addictions, even though their clients may be grappling with an addictive or semi-addictive issue and be too ashamed to bring it up. From my experience, many counselors and therapists seem to have been overly influenced by movies and TV. They see addictions as unsolvable problems and may even be afraid to treat "addicts."

Without realizing it, professionals seem to have an unconscious bias against anyone with an addictive issue. They may also have bought into the idea that addiction problems are distinctly different from any other problems someone comes to a counselor for. There are still inpatient facilities where treatment for addiction is separate from treatment for other psychological problems, as if one doesn't interact with the other. And they may think that "you have to be one to treat one." This is very unfortunate because most of my clients with addictive issues—and usually other issues, as well—are indistinguishable from any of my other clients. I'm sure my receptionist never knew who was there for depression, relationship problems, social anxiety, or an addiction.

Textbox 4.1. Case—Caroline: Friday and Saturday?!

"How much are you drinking?" I asked. Caroline had come to my office because she was concerned that she might be addicted to alcohol.

"About a half a bottle a day, but often I drink more than half."

"What? Wine, vodka, Scotch . . . ?"

"White wine."

Caroline was a professional accountant, a runner, and very slim.

"Well, more than a half a bottle—even a half a bottle—is quite a bit for a woman of your weight. What do you want to do in therapy?"

"Moderate."

At that time, Dr. Alan Marlatt, who created the concept of relapse prevention and, later, introduced the idea of harm reduction to this country, suggested that people who wanted to moderate should stop for a month. Then they could start again. When I suggested that, Caroline practically fell off the couch.

"I can see that that doesn't sound like a good idea to you. How about taking a week off?"

That also was met with a grimace.

"How about every other day?"

She brightened up. That seemed quite doable. But then she scowled a bit and asked, "Does that mean both Friday and Saturday?"

I smiled and said, "Yes, I think so, but you get to choose which day," and I thought to myself, she has much more of a problem than she realizes or is acknowledging.

She chose Friday.

Earlier I have discussed the importance of ongoing assessment in modern psychotherapy. Homework is very, very useful for that purpose. Here was a clear example. Her question, "Does that mean both Friday and Saturday?" gave me a much better idea about Caroline's drinking.

The following Tuesday, Caroline entered my office looking terrible. "I couldn't not drink one day of the entire week," she said, in a woeful tone. "I can't believe it. Even last night when I knew I was coming in to see you. What am I going to do? This is awful. Am I an alcoholic? I must be. I'm in such a mess. What can I do?"

Even though she may have failed at doing the homework, the homework had not failed. It had moved her from Stage II, Contemplation to Stage IV, Action, in one week.

Chapter 5

Step 3: Agree on the Therapeutic Goals

In a demonstration of DBT, Dr. Marsha Linehan said to her client: "So where do you want to go with all this hard work? If you say Boston and we see you driving off to Chicago, we'll know you're not going to get to where you said you want to go. We need to know where you want to go before we can tell whether you're on the right track." Many, many years before, I had read *Purposive Behavior in Animals and Men* (Tolman, 1951), because I could not buy into the theory that all human behavior could be explained by stimulus-response reinforcement, the dominant idea in American psychology in the 1960s. The author, Dr. Edward Tolman, and professor of psychology at UC Berkeley, argued that even rats created and used cognitive maps to find their way through a maze as quickly as possible, and his research studies made that clear. I was heartened to hear Linehan put such emphasis on purposeful goals. Where did her client want to go? In a somewhat similar manner, Hayes and ACT have put great emphasis on values and using values to guide one's life.

Modern therapy is future oriented and goal focused. In session, sometimes I think to myself, "Do I know the goals here?" If I don't, I wait until what seems like a good time, and say, "So, I'm not sure I know what your therapeutic goals are. What are we working toward?" Sometimes it helps to use prompts: "How would we know if therapy is working in three months? What would have changed?" It is important that we work with clients to identify reasonable emotional goals, behavioral goals, cognitive goals, interpersonal goals, existential/spiritual goals, and professional goals.

Recently, a client, Barbara, was telling me about everything that had gone wrong in her life. The list was long. Her stepfather had died six months ago, she had lost her job, her mother was ill. . . . Careful listening, as every therapist would agree, is terribly important in good therapy. But after 20 minutes, I raised my hands, made the time-out signal, and, after she had slowed down and stopped, I said, "That sounds really terrible, but what would you like to work on today?"

I subsequently learned that for Barbara, therapy was a place to vent. To some extent, past therapists had taught her this, so it was understandable. She did not have a narcissistic personality disorder, but she lived alone and had no one else to talk to. Her sister and friends didn't want to listen to her complain. Allowing her to continue to go on about the bad things in her life would not have helped her very much either. How could we help her break out of that pattern? What did she want to get out of therapy? What were her goals?

WHAT CAN YOU DO?

Behavioral Goals

Some people never want to have a panic attack again. Others want to be able to get done what they want to have done by the end of the day, a goal that consistently eludes them. I think of these as behavioral goals. Of course, if they behave better—"better" meaning more in line with their goals and values—they will feel better and they will think about themselves and their lives and their relationships in a very different manner. Everything affects everything.

Emotional Goals

Helping a client figure out how they could feel is an important part of modern therapy. If they have had a very critical parent and that parent is still very critical, how could they feel? This very idea, that one could intentionally aim to feel differently, may not make sense to some readers.

"I have a right to my feelings, don't I?" a client asked me during one of my first sessions as a therapist in training. We had not worked together long, and she had heard (incorrectly) that REBT therapists encouraged people to "just not feel."

"Of course, you do," I answered. "And feelings well up in us sometimes in ways that are really difficult to manage. But that's what you feel initially. I call that at Time 1. I don't know whether I would say you have a 'right' to your emotions, but you certainly have them at Time 1. And you have them whether you want them or not.

"If you want to stay angry, that's fine with me. Feeling very angry at times is not necessarily unhelpful. Some women don't let themselves feel angry. They have been socialized against expressing anger. Anxiety, shame, guilt, and depression are okay but not anger. If they even start to feel angry, they may feel panicky, hopeless, and trapped instead. But reasonable anger can help you get what you want. It's very empowering. Rage is another thing. Rage just makes everything worse. Rage is destructive.

"But what about at Time 2? You can have something to say about that. Let's assume you do not want to be so angry or enraged. Then what? How would you like to feel? You may not succeed completely, but it may be very helpful to talk about your options. Annoyed, irritated, aggravated, sad, resentful, regretful? Which makes sense to you?"

Helping a client be more specific and more realistic about their emotional goals can be very, very illuminating. When I ask, "How would you like to feel?" the client may say, "I want to feel better."

Then I may ask, "What does that mean?" I may also give them a list of emotional words to help them.

Sometimes during workshops, usually in the afternoon, at about 2:00 p.m., I ask people what they would like to feel at work. We put a list on the board:

happy
content
relaxed
valued
calm
challenged

validated
appreciated

Then I ask them to think about how they felt at 2:00 p.m. the previous day at work. We put that list on the board, too:

angry
irritated
tired
exhausted
anxious
not valued
unappreciated

The lists practically never overlap at all. Some of my clients deal with that problem by trying to numb themselves. Others smoke cigarettes or vape. Some use prescribed medications. What about you at work as a counselor or therapist? How would you like to feel when you are working during a session? Happy? Content? The meaning of those words differs significantly from person to person. Some practitioners think that what they are doing is too important to feel "happy" or "content" while doing it. Unfortunately, in English, there are not many words for the emotions we feel when we are focused, attentive, and engaged. I enjoy my work, but I am not "happy" at work. I have responsibilities. I must pay attention and listen carefully.

What could we feel? Fortunately, the inclusion of mindfulness into counseling and therapy offers an answer. We can feel grateful. We can feel grateful that we have or are about to have a license. We can help people and get paid to do so. We can be grateful that we have something engaging and challenging and often enjoyable to do in life. It isn't always easy given the conditions that some readers must work under, but we could feel grateful that we can learn and get better at what we do professionally.

"Grateful" works because you can be grateful and sad at the same time. You may be listening to someone telling you about being abused by a family member when they were seven. "Content," "happy," "satisfied," or "calm" don't fit the situation. Grateful, sad, regretful, and concerned are more appropriate. You can be grateful that the person survived and is trying to overcome the hurt and damage, and that you may be able to be of help.

You could also feel curious and open if you count those states of being as feelings. What might you learn from the next client or the next group you run? What might you learn from the next article or book you read or YouTube video you watch or workshop you attend?

Interpersonal Goals

William Glasser, the founder of reality therapy, asserted that everyone in your office, no matter what the complaint, was suffering from a relationship problem. A relationship had ended or was in danger of ending.

I agree. Most people are in my office because of interpersonal problems. They may say they are there because they are anxious or depressed or drinking too much, but if I scratch the surface, I often find that either a significant relationship is seriously in danger or has ended or they live alone and are miserably lonely.

Unfortunately, it is often easier to help someone stop using cocaine than to help them with a problem in a close, personal relationship. Relationships are very complex for many reasons.

First, they involve another person with their own values, likes and dislikes, quirks, personal plans and goals, and ideas about how a relationship "should" work. Each person also brings into the relationship baggage from earlier relationships, including, of course, our relationships with our original caregivers. Individuals may also bring into the relationship mood disorders, unique drives, or sleep issues. All of these can create challenges and be difficult to manage.

I sometimes joke that most gurus are not married and do not have children, and Epictetus and Epicurus both taught their students to stay clear of close relationships. Sex was okay, but close relationships would only lead to pain. In my opinion, they are both right and wrong. When a close relationship ends it is very painful for most people. Sometimes it takes years to recover. But close relationships can also be very enjoyable and, more importantly, they challenge us and help us grow.

Cognitive/Thinking Goals

Psychotic people clearly do not like the voices that they hear, but people who are not psychotic are also often troubled by the chatter in their heads. In fact, many people drink alcohol at the end of the day so as quiet their brain. There are at least two ways of thinking about this problem. One way notes that the client worries and ruminates all day and half the night. A second way considers the brain as the guilty party, not the person. Most of the time, their brain does what it is supposed to do. Feedback loops between their brain and their liver, lungs, stomach, gut, and thousands of muscles keep everything running smoothly. But did they pay the mortgage bill? Will they lose their job? Is their child very sick or just sick? The brain monitors everything, including that, and sometimes won't stop.

As I said in chapter 2, I like to suggest to clients that they have a "committee" upstairs with members who have different opinions and histories and hurts and fears and goals and values. Some psychologists and philosophers have suggested that these "voices" reflect different "selves," but this book is not based on that theory. Neuroscience research indicates that your client has thousands of neural networks whose jobs are to help you drink a cup of coffee without spilling, make sure the oxygen/carbon monoxide balance in your brain is okay, and worry about and make sure you pay the bills, do the laundry, and monitor the child coughing in the next room.

One of your client's "cognitive goals" may be to get the "committee" members to quiet down. But getting the committee to quiet down quickly or completely may not be a reasonable goal. And if your client thinks *I can't stand this anymore*, that will probably make things worse. It may help to accept that (1) Brains are supposed to work this way. (2) If your client's ancestors' brains had not worked this way, they might not be here: "Did you cut enough wood? Did you preserve enough fruit? Did you close the barn door?" People with brains like that probably lived longer and gave birth to more "little worriers" than those who did not have brains like that. (3) It is annoying, but there are things your client can do to help manage the problem, discussed throughout the book.

Sensory/Physical Goals

Before 1995, doctors assessed four "vital signs": temperature, pulse, respiration rate, and blood pressure. Then the president of the American Pain Society started to push the idea that doctors should also assess for pain, as a fifth vital sign. That opened a Pandora's box. Regardless of the ongoing controversy over this idea, many people suffer from pain and look for relief, as you know, often in opioids. Focusing on psychological goals and ignoring physical goals ignores that they interact. Physical goals may also include losing weight and/or exercising more, and we now know that exercising helps in the relief of many psychological ailments like anxiety and depression, as well as physical ailments.

Existential/Spiritual Goals

As I have noted earlier, humans live in time. Clients worry about the future and reflect on the past. And, as the existentialist and humanist psychologists have often reminded us, we die. The ACE study provides strong evidence that many people are significantly affected psychologically and physically by what happened in their childhood. But they may be even more affected by what they think about existential/spiritual issues (e.g., what they should have done in the past, what they should be doing now, and what they should do in the future).

Existentialism as a movement came out of WWI and II. Prior to WWI, war was not as horrible. Difficult as it may be to imagine, many men were excited about going to war in 1914, not knowing what lay ahead of them. The world had become industrialized and new, far more lethal methods of killing had been developed. The men who went to war and the cities and civilians in them were massacred in ways never before seen on the planet, culminating in the dropping of two atom bombs in WWII. Many people, not just existentialists, started to wonder: How could there be a god if such horror could occur? What is the meaning of existence, given what has happened? How can we find a meaningful way to live, given what is happening?

For some people, their religion and their saints and god or gods provide an answer to these questions. But even very religious people may be in your office grappling with them. Helping clients feel hopeful that they can find meaning and purpose in life may be one of the most important goals and outcomes of therapy.

Many ideas about spirituality are positive and hopeful, in line with the goals of most counselors and therapists. Psychotherapy and counseling have probably been influenced by William James's transcendentalist bias and Carl Roger's Protestant roots (i.e., each person finds their own path). However, Sollod (2005) correctly questions whether it is ethical for a therapist to nudge a client who holds more "hellfire and damnation" religious beliefs (e.g., the value of repentance and suffering, mortification of the flesh) toward more positive religious beliefs. He writes: "viewing spiritual health as necessarily compatible with psychological health is a naively selective view of the spiritual legacy of humanity" (p. 407).

This book does not encourage clinicians to push a particular stance vis-à-vis spirituality. However, if the client has found a practice or ritual helpful in the past, then the therapist may want to help the client restart it. Therapy, as advocated for in this book, is designed to help clients get back on track using a combination of activities, some of which are evidence-based, but some of which are not, at least, not yet.

In addition, this book does not see therapy as ever having as its primary focus and goal the spiritual development of the client. Most clinicians have not been trained as priests, ministers, rabbis, imams, or other kinds of spiritual leaders. Many traditional spiritual paths have leaders (Sollod calls them "spiritual directors") who explicitly tell initiates what to do and when. This is essentially a top-down model. The "master" knows what needs to be learned to successfully move along a particular spiritual path. As noted earlier, this book advocates for a collaborative, combined top-down/bottom-up model, in which the client ultimately decides what to do. However, that could include joining a cult-like religion or group. Sollod (2005) points out that "it is not difficult to find pseudo-Gnostic aspects of Freudian psychoanalysis, including its quasi-religious or cult-like organizational aspect, initiation through experience with a prior initiate, and the idea of hidden understandings open only to the correctly psycho-analyzed" (p. 408).

During the first group I ran with Ellis, at one point, I took the leap and said, "Well, as Dr. Ellis pointed out," and he cut me off. "Al! I don't want you to deify me like some other people seem to want to." I have known some very orthodox REBT-ers and CBT-ers over the years, but Ellis was not one of them, not even about REBT.

Drives and Needs

Oddly, many therapists, especially CBT-ers, hardly ever talk about drives, but some of the problems you encounter in your office may be the result of intense drives, for example, to create, to have sex, and/or to succeed. For the early psychoanalysts, drives were key, especially the sexual drive for Freud. Freud thought the sexual drive reflected a separate, distinct kind of energy, which he labeled the libido. No research has discovered such an energy, and energy is not yet the focus of much psychological research, but that doesn't mean that it doesn't play a significant role.

Alain de Botton, in his book *How to Think More about Sex* (2012), asks the question, What would life be like if we didn't have a sex drive? It's an intriguing question. Many people's lives would have been completely different. Asking about a client's sexual lives and fantasies is not required in many cases, but not asking may be a serious mistake with some clients. Marital relations are often greatly strained by differences in the drive for sex.

How are your client's goals affected by their innate drives? And does a drive create a "need"? If clients convince themselves that they absolutely have to have the love of another person or they absolutely must succeed or they need to be as thin as possible, serious trouble may follow.

There is no research evidence that one human's list is THE list of needs. Maslow's Hierarchy of Needs includes five: physiological (food and clothing), safety (job security), love and belonging (friendship), esteem, and self-actualization. There is also no research evidence that you cannot fill a need in the hierarchy unless you have fulfilled a lower need. For example, you can try to meet your need for love and belonging even if you have not met your physiological or safety needs. It is not, in fact, a hierarchy. Maslow's list has also been criticized as reflecting the needs of highly educated, privileged white males in an individualistic society but not the needs for many other people on the planet.

Glasser listed five needs: power, love and belonging, freedom, fun, and survival. For Rogers all humans strove for self-actualization but for Victor Frankl, the founder of logotherapy, humans needed to create meaning in life. After raising five children in multicultural New York City, sitting with clients for years, and observing humans in various cultures, my list includes:

1. Meaningful relationships, a feeling of belonging and of being connected
2. Safety
3. Meaningful work
4. Physical pleasure, including sex, eating, chilling, and doing what we like to do
5. Spiritual growth
6. The opportunity to learn

The drive to learn seems especially relevant to counseling and psychotherapy. As far as we can determine, no other organism on the planet decides to learn something new. Humans do so every day, from something relatively simple like a new dance or a new recipe to a new way of thinking about anxiety and/or the meaning of life. Our drive to learn seems innate. It may also be a result of our knowing that we exist in time and strongly desire to do something meaningful with our lives. The current focus on the brain, every day bringing us new insight into the functioning of the brain, is very exciting and may be useful in one or more ways in our practice, but it completely misses this most wonderful, unique aspect of humans. We love to learn and master new ways of thinking, feeling, and behaving, from tricycle riding to better ways to tolerate distress, frustration, and discomfort.

Chapter 6

Step 4: Set the Agenda

Very early in my career I asked a client, Ruth, the senior vice president of a large corporation in New York, "So what's on the agenda?" She immediately shot back, "I don't need agendas here. I have agendas up the wazoo in my office. I don't come here to talk about agendas."

I learned quickly that I had to be careful how I figured out what to focus on in a session. Clients often come to therapy to tell someone about their troubles and to find a sympathetic ear. However, solely listening for an entire session may not be very effective. (Of course, there are exceptions. If someone's partner has died, I'm probably going to sit and listen the entire session.)

Although Ruth didn't like the term "agenda," as a successful businesswoman, she did want to use her time wisely. We only had 50 minutes, and she only came once per week. I apologized and asked, "So how would you like to start?" I could have asked, "What would you like to work on?" but I thought that was also too close to her employment-related language.

When I worked as a consultant for the VA helping therapists become better at CBT for substance misuse, setting the agenda was the aspect of the program that they had the most difficulty doing. Many had been trained in a psychodynamic and/or a Rogerian approach. Neither approach advocates for a structured session or for setting an agenda.

We have discussed before that traditional talk therapy, especially psychoanalysis, was based on the theory that what is troubling your client is deeply buried and repressed in their unconscious. Consequently, it makes no sense to directly ask a client what they want to work on. The problem is too buried and defended against for them to answer such a question. In fact, psychodynamically trained therapists are quite sure that whatever a patient might say is the problem is definitely *not* the problem. As you can imagine, this not only might drive someone out of therapy, but it might also cause harm.

Rogers (1951) was one of the first psychologists to argue that people could identify their problems and articulate them, often in the first session. He didn't believe that the source of the problem was so repressed and defended against that a client couldn't tell a therapist what was wrong. For that reason, Rogers named his form of therapy "client-centered," subsequently "person-centered." The client should and could guide the therapy. His was a bottom-up model in contrast to the-doctor-knows-best, top-down, medical model. And one of the guiding principles of this book is that therapy should be client centered.

But Rogers's therapy was a distinctly nondirective therapy. He didn't believe in guiding (directing) the therapy or the client in any way. Hence, no agenda. As a therapist, I know how easy it is to just listen. Anyone who has a good friend or partner has experienced how helpful it is simply to tell someone else who is supportive and caring about an issue. Talking does help. We may not understand why, but that is undeniably true.

However, therapy costs clients time and money, and most clients only come once a week or less. Then the question becomes, how can we work most efficiently? How can we best help our clients? Discussing the agenda and what a client wants to work on are important parts of the answers to those questions. Without some idea of what we are working toward and how we are going to use the 50 minutes that we have, we may waste a client's time.

It is important to note that some clients may have no interest in working "efficiently." Therapy costs very little or nothing for them, and they enjoy talking about their problems—for example, how unfair someone was to them in the past week. They like having their problems be the focus of attention and someone being attentive to them. Not many people outside of the therapist's office will be. However, that kind of behavior can strain if not destroy other relationships. Just listening by a therapist may reinforce this behavior. Eventually, even the therapist may start complaining about how narcissistic their client is, but they are partly responsible. Their behavior encouraged the client to talk about what happened in the past week.

I sometimes joke that there are three kinds of therapy: (1) Venting, which I'm fine with if someone has just had something terrible happen in their life, but not if I'm the third therapist they've talked about it with. I may let them vent, but not for very long. If it were curative, I would, but it is not. (2) Chatting, which is also fine for a while, and you can get paid for it! However, it can become dangerously close to the oldest profession in the world. Clients pay you money, and you give them lots of attention and make them feel better. (3) Goal-focused therapy—this is the form of therapy and counseling advocated for in this book, and setting the agenda often leads to a better session.

Chapter 7

Step 5: In-Session Work

It is relatively easy to do what I call empathy and encouragement therapy (EET): *"Oh, I am sorry to hear that. Tell me more about that."* and then, *"Well, I'm sure if we continue to work together, you will feel and do better."* Therapists and counselors can sit in their chairs and say things like that. They can see eight or 10 clients a day, and they don't have to stay up on the research to do that. But we can do better than EET. That is a major goal of this book.

What should you do as the fifth step and perhaps most important part of a session? Traditional therapy relies on the idea that insight into the cause—the "why?"—of the problem coupled perhaps with Rogerian unconditional regard, will be sufficient. But modern therapists are equally or perhaps more interested in "how?": How might the client do and feel better in the week ahead? As much time or more may be spent helping clients answer questions such as "Why do I feel this way?" "Why is this happening to me?" "Why do I keep acting this way?"

WHAT CAN YOU DO?

Restart Something That Has Helped in the Past

When Asha came into my office, she was depressed. Her boyfriend of five years had left her, and, at 37, she was worried that she might never have children, something that she wanted very much. She had also recently started a new job, which added to her stress.

It turned out that she had practiced a form of Pilates before. Research (Aibar-Almazán et al., 2019) indicates that Pilates is helpful in many ways, but like many people who have done something like Pilates, tai chi, or yoga and found it to be helpful, she did not know why she had stopped.

"Do you think you could start again?"

She seemed very open to the idea.

"How often did you go?"

"Twice a week."

"When would you do it now?" I asked. Research into implementation intentions (Gollwitzer & Sheeran, 2006). suggests that if you can help people specify when and where they are going to do something, they have a better chance of actually doing it. Specifically, if you can help them construct sentences like, "After I get up, I will meditate." Or "Once I have my coffee, I will start writing," there is a greater likelihood that they will do what they intend to do.

"Probably on Saturdays and one other time during the week," she answered.

"Where would you go?"

"Where I used to go."

"So, this is something you think will help and you seem open to doing. Is there anything that might derail this plan?"

"I don't think so."

"Maybe you might say, 'I'm too depressed to do Pilates today' or something like that?"

"No. I don't think so," she answered. The very idea seemed to have lifted her spirits. Here was something she could do. She could not make her ex-boyfriend stay with her and have a child. In fact, she didn't even want to do that. But when she started the session, she was feeling trapped, angry, hopeless, and helpless. Now there was something she could do, and it had helped in the past.

In this case, she did start going to two Pilates classes per week. In and of itself, that would not have been sufficient, but therapy plus Pilates plus better sleep helped her succeed in her new job and take the next necessary steps in her life.

Identify "Brain Lies," and Help Your Client Manage Them

Dr. Laurie Santos, professor of psychology at Yale University, who teaches the largest undergraduate course ever at Yale, "The Science of Well-Being" (also available on Coursera), says, "The brain lies." As I discussed in chapter 2, we have a lot of neural modular networks. They are wonderful. They monitor how our heart is functioning, help us walk straight and keep us inhaling and exhaling enough so that we don't die. I like to refer to them as "the Committee." Without them, we would not be able to function. However, some of them toss up ideas that are distinctly not helpful. Many readers are familiar with voices, not psychotic voices, that say things like, "You can't do this," when, in fact, they have done it successfully many times before. But that voice still chimes in. It's not true. It's a lie.

Some people who have problems with overeating may hear a voice say something like, "It's okay. I'll eat less tomorrow." This would be fine if it weren't a lie. They will very probably *not* eat less tomorrow.

People who have a problem with alcohol may hear a voice say, "A drink will make you feel better," which is not a lie, if you count only the short term. They may also hear a voice say, "I'll just have two." Past experience—often many, many past experiences—suggests that this is a lie. They will not "just" have two.

Clients who procrastinate hear, "I'll do it tomorrow." Or "I'll do it tomorrow when I feel better." Both are often or almost always lies.

Some of the automatic thoughts that the brain or the committee tosses up have no merit whatsoever. In fact, unfortunately, they may undermine your client's efforts to change: *You can't change. Nobody really changes.* Fortunately, these are lies.

Therapists can help clients recognize and accept that their brains, while doing many wonderful things for them, also occasionally lie. They can help clients accept that this is quite normal in human brains. Hating themselves for having such thoughts or trying to exorcize them completely will probably be a waste of time and energy. Shaming and blaming make no sense whatsoever and help not at all. Saks, who uses a combination of strategies to manage her schizophrenia, sees her negative voices as essentially frightened. She talks to them in a gentle, calming way, assuring them that she has taken care of them (and herself) in the past, and she is going to do so again.

Most people equate their brains with their selves. They do not see their brain as an organ that may, at times, malfunction. A depressed client once said to me, "I just thought, 'I can't do that,' and went to bed." I suggested that one part of his brain tossed up the ideas, *"I can't do that. I'm too tired to do that."* Then I asked, "Were there any other voices in your head?"

"Well, I knew I shouldn't go back to bed. Things always get worse when I go back to bed."

"So at least one member of your committee tried to object?"

"Yes."

"If other members spoke up, what do you think they would say?"

"'You can do that.' It was an email I was trying to write. I have written similar emails without any problem thousands of times. Often I say to myself, 'You don't feel well, but you can do it, and you will feel better when you do it.' Which is true. But yesterday I just couldn't get myself to do it."

"So your brain tossed up an idea totally without merit. You could have done it. Your brain, or at least a part of your brain, lied."

"Well, maybe. But why do I always give in? Why did I go back to bed?"

"That's a good question. Do you always give in when your brain tosses up a lie?"

"No."

"What made yesterday different?"

"It was a very gray day and what Trump said was so depressing. I just felt overwhelmed."

"Yes. That's understandable. We'll work together so that you just feel 'whelmed,' which is actually an English word, and not *over*whelmed. And we'll help you learn how to deal with brain lies."

DIY, In-the-Moment Therapy

In 1955, Ellis created his ABC model so that people could do therapy by themselves between sessions, in the moment, when life was happening. He also wanted a mnemonic that people could remember; hence, ABC. Currently, as I discussed in chapter 4, the ABC model is used in session to help clients and therapists conceptualize what is happening. It is also a standard form of between-session work (or "homework").

CBT (and REBT before it) became popular forms of therapy partly because they are so user-friendly. People can quite quickly understand them. We all know that we think irrational or unhelpful thoughts at times during the day. Learning how to manage such thoughts with in-the-moment techniques makes people feel more hopeful and empowered.

According to researchers Clark and Rhyno (2005), everyone engages in self-talk, most of it spontaneous but some of it goal directed. Their research also suggests that we have approximately 4,000 thoughts per day. Some of them are intrusive and unwanted. They pop up "out of nowhere." They affect how we feel and think and behave. ACT (along with Buddhism) suggests that our brain tosses up such thoughts as part of its ongoing monitoring of our internal systems and the external environment, including possible future environments: *Am I developing symptoms of a strange illness? OMG!*

Thirty years ago, when I first went to the then-named Institute for Rational Emotive Therapy, I was disdainful of the ABC technique. I was probably somewhat of a Manhattan, psychodynamic snob. How could lining up one of my 25 different, interacting problems help? It was too simplistic. It was even stupid, I thought, to think something like that.

However, I had an anger management problem. I was not in therapy at the time, so I did an ABC(DE) on my own, and it helped. The next time I got angry, I did another one. It also helped. Eventually, I probably did 200, sometimes on the forms the institute provided for free but at other times just on a piece of paper or the computer. Soon I could do them in my head.

Doing an ABC helps us gain insight into the ways we are thinking that make a bad situation worse. The first part of the ABC technique is the diagnostic part. (If you are new to the ABC technique, you can download forms and learn about them and how to use them by going online.) Doing an ABC with clients is designed to help clients gain insight into the ways they, themselves, contribute to a problem.

A: The Activating Event or Adversity

Many good therapists start with the A. They prefer to find out more about the situation. Traditional therapy spends a great deal of time talking about and focusing on the A, sometimes the entire session. That is not usually the best use of a client's time or money. It is far more important to gain insight into the Bs, the beliefs about the As.

B: The Beliefs about the A That Contribute to the C

The underlying theory to the ABC technique is new to many people. They think in terms of an A–C, causative connection: My boss yelled at me (the A) and that made me angry (the C). The ABC model suggests something quite different. You may believe and think to yourself something like: *A boss should never yell at an employee. It is so unprofessional! My boss hates me. I can't stand this. I have to get out of here.* It is your beliefs *about* your boss's yelling that creates your anger and contributes to your leaving the office. The Buddha 2,500 years ago said much the same thing and so did the Greek philosopher Epictetus: "People are not disturbed by things, but by the views they take of them."

C: The Consequence

I like to start at the C, the consequence, and work back in time. What contributed to making the C difficult and upsetting? For example, if a client is very anxious or depressed or if they had a nasty fight with their partner or they stayed up half the night binge watching a new series, what contributed, in terms of their thinking, to that happening? (Note: Occasionally a consequence can be a form of thinking, for example, ruminating or intrusive thoughts, delusions, and hallucinations.)

You can start at the A or the C. Both ways have merit. Neither is right nor wrong. Do what you feel comfortable doing but move on to the Bs fairly quickly.

Some clients have already read books or online articles about CT and CBT, and they like the model. The idea that they can have some control over their thinking, emoting, and behaving deeply appeals to them. But some clients come to our offices not knowing anything about this model. You can imagine the impact on such a client if you introduced the model by saying, "Well, of course, it is not what your boss said that is upsetting you; *you* are upsetting yourself about what she said." That comes very close to blaming the victim and may drive the client out the door.

Working in a more Rogerian way may help you introduce the model: "So your boss called you out in front of your coworkers, and then you got so enraged that you stormed out of the office. Do I have that right?" (Rogerian and MI-style reflective listening.)

"Yup. I know it was stupid, but I can't believe that he did that. It's so unprofessional."

"And now he's written something up and put it in your file because you left the office."

"Yes. It's so unfair. I work hard. I do my work well. He's just impossible."

"Yes. That's does seem very difficult. But what do you think you were thinking or 'telling yourself'—which is the way we talk about it here—to make yourself so very angry?"

Then watch your client carefully. How did they take that idea? Did it annoy them, or do they now seem more curious to figure this out? You may want to explicitly ask at the beginning of the next session something like, "I'm curious. How did you feel last session when I suggested that it was what you were thinking that contributed to your getting so angry and storming out of the office? Did that suggestion annoy you last session?"

Looking for the Bs—the helpful/rational and unhelpful/irrational beliefs, cognitive distortions, and brain lies—helps clients with five key insights:

1. The ABC model clearly signals that in your opinion and based on your model, it is not solely the activating event (the A) that is affecting them. It is their beliefs about the A— their demandingness, inflexibility, awfulizing, and brain lies—that play a key role in how they feel and behave. They may not be able to change what is happening outside of them, but they can work on managing their emotional and behavioral reactions better.
2. Some beliefs are flexible and helpful and make everything work better. In contrast, some beliefs are rigid, inflexible, and unhelpful and make everything worse.
3. Some beliefs are simply lies.
4. Some events lead to appropriate ("appropriate" in the sense that they fit the situation) but negative and often unpleasant emotions. Sometimes trying to change those negative emotions just because clients don't like them will work against their long-run goals and values.
5. Humans can have a combination of emotions at the same time. They can feel very sad and anxious about losing their temper and grateful about something else (e.g., that their daughter did well in soccer).

What is the problem with the model? To a client, it may suggest that if they have a problem—they are depressed because they are unemployed and may lose their home—they should just change their thinking. It does not honor that external factors may play a significant role. Carol Graham, a senior fellow at the Brookings Institute, points out that the loss of manufacturing jobs in the United States has contributed to widespread feelings of despair, especially among middle-aged men in that area. The ABC model may suggest that nothing outside them needs fixing. They need fixing, which is, again, blaming the victim.

On the other hand, thinking that they are doomed, helpless, and hopeless does not help either. Fortunately, they can do both: Work to change the system as they work to change how they may disempower themselves with unhelpful, irrational thinking.

D: Disputing (or Questioning as an Alternative to Disputing)

Albert Ellis grew up in a very stimulating, Jewish neighborhood in the Bronx. We have Hitler to thank for that. Some of the brightest minds in Europe moved to the States and settled in that area. Ellis grew up with other teenagers who loved to argue about all sorts of philosophical and political ideas. Nine students from the high school in that neighborhood went on to win Nobel prizes in science.

In the ABCDE model, the D stands for dispute, and fits very nicely with ABC. ABCD! I prefer to pick a belief or automatic thought and question its validity or helpfulness or merit. But that may be because I don't like to debate or "dispute." Of course, ABCQ is not as memorable as ABCD.

In the early days of Ellis's form of CBT, REBT, the therapist or the client was supposed to dispute the irrational beliefs of the client. In fact, in the first half of his career, Ellis was very disputatious, and many professionals found it extremely off-putting. Research suggests that being argumentative and disputatious with a client is generally ineffective and may even make matters worse. But Ellis served up his confrontive, very New York style therapy with empathy, a huge smile, and a great deal of humor. Occasionally, in the past, at the institute, but, fortunately, not now, I would pass a therapy room and hear a young therapist arguing with a client. That kind of behavior on the part of a therapist may have happened because young therapists, watching Ellis work with clients during a Friday night demonstration, could not see the way Ellis was also strongly empathic and supportive. Ellis never argued with clients. He tried to help them argue with the irrational beliefs that supported their inflexible, rigid thinking.

How quickly should you move from collecting the A, B, and C to the D and E? That is not possible to answer. Every individual client and session is different. But it is very important to move on to the D and E. Those parts may be the most therapeutic part of the ABCDE model.

All Ds are questions:

Where is the evidence that your boss hates you?
How does thinking that way help?
What do you mean by "I can't stand it anymore?"

Such questions are a form of what Beckian-trained therapists refer to as Socratic questioning. The D portion helps clients question the validity or helpfulness or merit of one or more of their Bs. You can find many different forms of the ABC online and people do an ABC in many different ways, but the original and best form includes the D.

Questions, either by a therapist or on the part of someone doing an ABCDE on their own, bring insight into the kind of thinking, feelings, behaviors, and interpersonal difficulties that may be making the situation worse. They may also reveal how rigidly clients are holding on to their beliefs.

Working therapeutically in a session is an art. Sometimes it is helpful to be Socratic in one's approach. But there are times when some clients benefit from a more direct, didactic approach. For someone grappling with depression, if I think it is true, I may say, "I think you might be saying something to yourself like 'I can't stand it' or 'It won't matter.'"

Many therapists do not use the ABC technique at all, and there are clients that I don't use it very often with either. However, especially if you run groups, it is a very powerful technique to learn, but it is one of the most difficult to learn to do well. The VA in its CBT program for substance disorders skipped the D part and moved straight to the E. But with some clients, this part is well worth the time and effort to perfect.

E: More Effective Thoughts, Feelings, and Behaviors

Part E helps clients develop another kind of insight. You can do it in session if you have time or you can give the client an ABCDE worksheet and ask them to fill it in on their own and bring it back to the next session.

> *What could you think instead? (or have thought instead?)*
>> My boss doesn't hate me. He just doesn't always control his temper, the way I would like him to.
>> I don't always get things the way I want.
>> I don't like that kind of behavior, but I can stand it.
>> Thinking about looking for another job is also a possibility.
>> I'm not a failure just because I ran out of the office.
>
> *What could you feel instead? (or have felt instead?)*
>> Annoyed, sad, regretful. (Some people do, in fact, have better bosses.)
>> Grateful. (I have a job. Most of the time he likes my work.)
>> Determined. (To behave better in the future).

Hopeful. (I can learn to handle bad situations like this without behaving badly myself.)
What could you do instead? (or have done instead?)

Leave the situation but not the office.

Practice with my therapist—role play—learning to behave more assertively when someone attacks me. For example, I can learn to ask questions instead of just freezing.

Call a friend.

Deep breathe and listen to my meditation app.

Cognitive Defusion

Like DBT, acceptance and commitment therapy (ACT) emphasizes the importance of mindfulness. Hayes theorizes that language and the way humans react to linguistic ideas are the basis of human suffering. Moreover, humans get beliefs "fused" to their sense of self, to their identities, leading them to hold onto those ideas in a rigid, non-flexible way.

Hayes strongly asserts that questioning (disputing) such ideas or beliefs will only strengthen them. You are giving meritless ideas some legitimacy. In place of questioning/disputing beliefs, ACT encourages clients to practice "cognitive defusion." Such exercises are designed to help someone become less identified with and attached to their thoughts. Clients can learn many techniques to facilitate cognitive defusion (see Hayes & Smith, 2005, pp. 83–84, for a list). For example, some clients find it helpful to imagine putting one of their thoughts on a leaf and letting it gently drift away down a quiet stream.

You can encourage clients to say to themselves, "I notice the thought," or "Thank you, brain, for that thought." This is similar to when I suggest to a client that "a member of your committee" (see chapter 2) is tossing up a thought that may have no merit at all. Instead of "I can't do it," they can think "Some part of my brain is suggesting that I can't do it." Thinking in this manner *about* their thoughts may help them identify less with them and become less fused with them and more psychologically flexible.

Defusion or Disputing or Both?

You will no doubt discover that some clients like one approach (examining and questioning the validity and helpfulness of their thoughts), other clients prefer the other (just letting such thoughts go), and some use both. When they are angry at someone, they may discover, perhaps having done an ABC in their head or on paper, that they are creating the anger by thinking something like *He should not have said what he said. It is so unfair and unjust considering everything I have done.*

Possibly, they can simply let such thoughts go because getting angry—any kind of anger—might not be in line with their goals and values. However, letting go of such thoughts can be extremely difficult because we deeply believe what we believe: *My boss should not behave unprofessionally!* It sounds completely reasonable and rational. No doubt, letting go of such thoughts/beliefs would be very helpful. But questioning the validity of a thought will not always strengthen it. In fact, it may be of value to examine the rationality and/or helpfulness of such a thought. Moreover, it may be easier for clients to let go of such thoughts after examining them. They can then see that (1) they have irrational components (e.g., *I can't stand being yelled at. A boss must always behave the way I think they should behave*) and (2) holding onto and thinking such thoughts won't help them fulfill their goals.

In his TED Talk (2016, https://www.youtube.com/watch?v=o79_gmO5ppg), Hayes clearly did not simply let go of the beliefs that had plagued him. Ultimately, his technique was a

Textbox 7.1. Case—Tony's Rule # 1: A Man Must Always Do a Good Job

Recently, a client, Tony, and I were working together, and we gained insight into the fact that he had a "rule" (CBT-ers say a "belief" or "automatic thought," but with some clients, the word *rule* seems to work better.): *A man must always do a good job.*

Of course, such a rule might be helpful if it is not held rigidly and in an absolutistic, perfectionist manner. In a less rigid form, you can hold it as a guiding principle: "Always try to do things well," by which you mean, "as well as you can at that moment." But his rule seemed to be: "I must always do things well or I'm not a real man." With his rule, he had suffered from persistent depressive disorder (PDD), in the past called "dysthymia" (low-grade chronic depression), and anxiety almost all of his life.

I asked Tony, "How do you think you got that rule? And when?"

He was quite clear: from his mother. Freud is smiling. According to Jake, his mother had raised him by using guilt and shame as the way to control him, his brother, and his sister. His mother did not hit them. But she was a perfectionist. His father had died when he was seven, so whatever he believed about what it meant to be a man he had to learn from his environment without a father.

Tony had always done well in school, unlike his two siblings. He had been president of his senior high school class and gone on to an Ivy League university. An MBA followed from another prestigious East Coast university, and now he was a project manager for a large real estate company. He was a highly valued employee. He was also a good father, husband, friend, and son. But he constantly worried and several (nonpsychotic) voices in his head were never satisfied and always critical: He was not doing enough *to be a real man.*

Tony recognized that he had overlearned the rule. Years of conditioning by his mother and by himself on himself had, in a sense, cemented the rule into his brain.

We had uncovered the "rule" doing an ABC in my office. I have no doubt that another therapist might have gotten the same results by simply asking, "What rule do you think you might be following in your life that drives you to overwork?" Or they might have asked the Miracle Question (from solution-focused therapy): "If you woke up tomorrow morning and all of your anxiety and depression were completely, miraculously gone, what would be different about your day?" There are many ways to help clients gain insight into their own particular ways of thinking and behaving that contribute to their problems.

In this case, insight helped immensely. He had a clue into why he constantly overworked, according to him and corroborated by his wife. But insight would not be enough. He had to chip away at the problem from several different directions, cognitively, emotively, behaviorally, interpersonally, and, as he was a practicing Catholic, spiritually.

behavioral one, very similar to the one Ellis frequently told to explain how he overcame his fear of speaking to women. Hayes lets go of his belief that it would be "awful" if he failed, but no one can know if he also, at some point in time, examined or questioned the rationality of *If I fail, it will be awful*. He says that he talked with his wife about his fear. Perhaps she suggested it was irrational. Perhaps talking to his wife was the therapeutic key. Without it, he could not have let go of the thought.

Hayes also believes that looking for the reason behind feelings and thoughts is counterproductive. But he appears to have looked for the reasons behind his fears. He tells his TED Talk viewers that he realized that what was happening triggered thoughts (and perhaps images?) of terribly scary times as a child. But then he advocates for simply letting those thoughts go. I cannot see the advantage of not using both techniques—plus other techniques that increase insight into what is going on—which is what Hayes appears to have done, at least based on what he says in his talk.

Ignoring unhelpful thoughts may work well when your client wants to have done something (e.g., have gone to the gym). Most of us do not like to go to the gym. Quite often, prior to going to the gym, a variety of distinctly unhelpful thoughts may go through our heads: *You could go tomorrow. You have a lot to do today. You're tired. Why not go tomorrow?* If your client pays any attention to such thoughts, the thoughts may get stronger, and if they engage in a debate, they may notice that they *always* lose. They don't go to the gym. So successfully going to the gym may involve letting go of certain thoughts that the brain tosses up without entertaining them or questioning them. Going is in line with their goals and values. Hence, as ACT suggests, using a cognitive defusion technique will work better.

In a similar way, a client of mine found cognitive defusion helpful for dealing with his psychotic thoughts: *That man following me is a CIA agent.* Learning to identify such thoughts and then learning to let them go as having no merit was exceptionally helpful. But how did he arrive at the idea that the FBI-agent image had no merit? Questioning the rationality and helpfulness of such a belief may also have been helpful. In summary, there are times when a cognitive defusion technique may work better for a client than examining and questioning a belief, but there also may be times when the reverse may be true. Most importantly, you can urge clients to discover what works best for them in what situations and with which beliefs.

Mindfully Managing Perceptions, Interpretations, and Evaluations

Let's imagine a possible scenario: A high school junior, Jim, walks into a meeting of the student council, and, according to him, no one says hello. In fact, a friend, Kaitlyn, does say hello, but he doesn't notice. His interpretation of what is happening is as follows: *No one said hello. I don't fit in here. No one really likes me.* Imagine that at the time, Jim is going to an almost all white high school, and he is non-white, so some of these thoughts may not be irrational. However, it is his evaluations more than his interpretations that may create real trouble: *This is awful. I can't stand it. I have to get out of here.* The accompanying emotions and physical sensations? Probably some combination of shame, anger, rage, humiliation, and/or anxiety.

It is important to notice that if he didn't evaluate/rate what he thought was going on so negatively, he would not have had that kind of reaction. If he had just observed his interpretations, he would have remained calmer. Of course, that's very difficult for most people, especially for teenagers.

Fortunately, clients can learn to observe more mindfully. First, they can learn to be more careful about how they perceive what is going on. Jim didn't perceive the situation correctly at the very beginning. Someone had, in fact, said hello. Then they can learn to be more careful about how they interpret what they perceive. Finally, they can be much more careful about how they rate or evaluate their interpretations. This has been a major aspect of DBT, ACT, and other mindfulness-based therapies. It may take years of practice, and good teachers and therapists can be extraordinarily helpful along the way.

Judging and Rating

Humans judge and rate everything, all the time, including their behaviors and, often, their "self." It is not the ratings in and of themselves that are the problem. It is the way that a client rates or judges everything and how they interpret and evaluate that rating that may cause difficulties. Specifically, they may jump to global judgments of the entirety of themselves, others, or life and the world. It is that jump that creates problems. If someone lies to your client, they may tell you, "He lied." But they may also be thinking, "and he's a shit. I hate him." If your client is talking about themselves, the same dynamic may be at work: *I lied. I'm a liar* (as if they always lied) *and I'm a shit. I hate myself.*

Rating and evaluating can lead to serious problems, especially when it involves oneself and others. It is impossible to evaluate the entirety of a person accurately and correctly. They are too complex. Human neurochemistry and behavior also change from minute to minute and situation to situation. Moreover, what one person may like in a particular person, another may detest. Not everyone will agree on any evaluation as to its accuracy or correctness.

Deep Diaphragmatic Breathing

Deep diaphragmatic breathing (DDB) is a relatively quick and easy technique that your client can use in the moment to manage spikes in their anxiety and prevent panic attacks. It effectively tricks the brain into releasing neurochemicals to help clients calm down. Teaching clients how to do it in session and checking the next few sessions, as any good coach would do, will help them learn to better manage their anxiety.

We are stuck in mammalian bodies. It is in our mammal nature to freeze, run, or fight when faced with real or imagined danger. When we get stressed, our diaphragm tightens up, and we begin to breathe in a shallower manner. Our brain takes this as a signal of danger and starts to pump adrenalin, cortisol, and other neurochemicals into our system.

We can reverse this vicious feedback loop by breathing deeply, so deeply that our diaphragm relaxes and goes down. This tricks the brain into thinking that the danger has gone. Then it starts sending out calming neurochemicals, such as gamma-aminobutyric acid (GABA), glutamate, and serotonin.

You can teach a client or a group how to do DDB quite easily. Ask your client or group members to do the following: "Put your right hand on your chest and your left hand on your stomach/gut. Breath in slowly. Counting slowly—1, 2, 3, 4, 5—may help you."

Count with them, slowly.

"Which hand moved? If your right hand moved, that means that you breathed into your chest and did not relax your diaphragm. Breath in slowly again. This time, try to make sure that your left hand—the hand on your stomach/gut—moves out but your right hand doesn't move at all."

Count again, slowly.

"If your left moved out and not your right, you have successfully breathed in deeply. Now breath out again to the count of five. Do it again. Some people like to hold their breath for five before they exhale and before they inhale. This is called 'box breathing.'"

DDB is an example of what I call "body work." It may be much more effective than any cognitive approach. That is, DDB may be much more helpful to your clients than saying to themselves, "Calm down. It's not the end of the world. Relax." Initially, it may be difficult for some clients to learn, and others may dismiss it as too simple to be helpful, but it is the quickest, most effective, least expensive way to reduce anxiety.

An Integrated, Culturally Sensitive Approach

Most people resolve the difficulties that they face in life on their own, without professional help. Of course, as we know, that is not true for everyone. The suicide rate continues to rise in the United States and accidental overdoses now exceed deaths from automobile accidents. But most people get better on their own. Many people also live long lives while managing life-threatening diseases such as diabetes, lupus, and AIDS.

How do they do it?

They do it by combining a number of strategies. If you had COVID, I'm sure that you tried to drink more liquids—maybe you were lucky and someone (or you) made chicken soup for you—rested more, and perhaps took aspirin, Tylenol, and/or an ibuprofen. If you were worried about getting really sick, you may have also seen a doctor or gone to the emergency room. Some of you prayed and some made an offering of some kind or did some other kind of religious ritual. You may have also bought an oximeter. Former president Trump was reportedly given eight drugs when he was hospitalized.

To manage panic attacks, people often combine a number of techniques, although they may not be aware that they are doing so. They may go to a psychiatrist, who will prescribe an SSRI (e.g., Paxil, Zoloft) or a SNRI (e.g., Effexor), or a benzodiazepine such as Xanax or Klonopin. And they may go to a counselor or other form of psychotherapist, and depending on the therapist's training, they will either look for the causes of the panic attacks in their past or in what they are thinking about current situations. In addition, they may go online or read a book (or reread sections of a book that has helped them in the past), reduce their caffeine intake, start or restart using some form of meditation app, try to get more sleep, and start or restart some form of exercise. Using a combined approach, they can greatly reduce the number and severity of panics attack or never have them again.

People also use a combination and a variety of ways to manage addictions. Therapy and groups may help them reframe the problem as a serious, risky health behavior rather than a behavior that they have to be ashamed of. No one gets in trouble with an addiction saying to themselves, *I think I'll take X (or do X) and make my life much more difficult.* It happens inadvertently and accidently. But once people have become addicted to one or more chemicals or behaviors, to change that or those behaviors and to maintain the change or changes requires a combination of strategies, perhaps including, depending on the individual, self-help groups, meditation, prayer, individual and group therapy, bibliotherapy, exercise, medication, and perhaps even intensive inpatient treatment (i.e., rehab). The majority of the participants in my SMART Recovery groups use seven to eight strategies. Some use fifteen. Of course, the same is true if you have another serious health issue, such as cancer, diabetes, or a cardiac problem. You will use a combination of strategies to try to stay well.

Chapter 8

Step 6: Agree on Between-Session Work

Early in his career, Ellis came up with an idea that was radical at that time: Clients could and should do therapy on themselves between sessions. Most clinicians laughed at the idea. It ran completely counter to everything that they had been taught. Clients (patients, for them, most of whom were doctors) could only make progress while in their offices, when slips of the tongue, dreams, and so on, could be analyzed. Consequently, many patients went five times a week; some went more. Psychoanalysis was and is a strongly top-down model, and, according to the model, the patient cannot overcome their defenses and work on their problems on their own.

Ellis thought otherwise, and perhaps the biggest change in psychotherapy over the past 50 years has been the recognition of the significant value of between-session work. (Cooper et al., 2017; Decker et al., 2016; Kazantzis et al., 2016; Mausbach et al., 2010). At times, and with some issues, the processing and practice that occurs between sessions may be more important than what occurs in session.

Ideally, something during the session will suggest a good between-session activity for your client to engage in. But if that doesn't happen, the last part of a session should be devoted to discussing what might be helpful to do between sessions. It may be one, two, or even a number of things, such as listening to an app, starting to meditate again, doing an ABC worksheet, going to a meeting, making an appointment with a psychiatrist, and/or baking banana bread.

Almost all between-session assignments can work even when they may appear not to have worked. I learned that in my first year at the institute. My goal for the first session was to help my client move from one stage to the next in the Stages of Change model. Caroline (see the case in chapter 4) came into the office wondering whether she had a drinking problem. The homework moved her from contemplation to action in one week.

Between-session work is designed with six key objectives for the client:

1. Observing and gaining increased insight into the difficulties they are grappling with
2. Observing and gaining insight into what helps manage those problems
3. Learning to be more accepting of discomfort and frustration, both often felt when trying new behaviors
4. Learning to deal effectively with experiential avoidance
5. Increasing hope and motivation by experiencing one's own agency or self-efficacy: *I can do it, and I did it*
6. Practicing being more self-compassionate regarding their selves and their ups and downs, successes and failures

Occasionally, you may come up with something to do during the coming week right after the check-in. But if you don't watch the clock, it's very easy for the session to end and you have not agreed on any between-session work. Consequently, when something during the session suggests it, I try to discuss what might work as between-session "homework" right then and there. In fact, the best form of between-session work seems to come up in a natural way during the in-session work. But if it does not, you need to stop five minutes early to discuss what might be helpful between sessions.

I put an HA with a circle around it next to what we have agreed upon in my notes. That makes it easier to remind myself before the next session what we had agreed to do. HA stands for "homework assigned"; you might like the Beck Institute's term, action plan, and use an AP with a circle around it. The point is to make it clear in your notes what you have agreed upon and not to forget to ask about how it went.

WHAT CAN YOU DO?

Have Your Client Restart Something That Has Helped Them in the Past

As noted in chapter 7, you can often help clients feel and get better very rapidly by getting them to restart what has helped them in the past. Some may say, "That's not therapy." But how is that true if doing so is very therapeutic? If your client starts to do again what has helped in the past, they may feel and do better very quickly and then decide to do some deeper therapy with you. Unfortunately, it is quite typical of humans to start to practice an exercise routine and, when they're feeling better, to gradually stop. Then, when they are not feeling well, they often don't start it up again—whatever "it" is—without a nudge. In the previous chapter, I shared how Asha had found it very helpful to start Pilates again.

Meditation and Prayer

There are many forms of meditation. That a client may have tried one form and it didn't seem to help doesn't mean that there isn't another form that they would find very helpful and agreeable to include in their busy daily schedule.

According to the Dalai Lama:

> In my own practice, I engage mostly in analytical meditation. This is a form of mental investigation where you can see your thoughts as thoughts and learn not to be chained to them, not to identify with them. You come to recognize that your thoughts do not necessarily reflect the truth. In analytical mediation, you are constantly asking, What is reality? What is that self, or "I," that we hold so dear and is the focus of so much of our concern?
>
> Some forms of meditation are just trying to create a state of thoughtlessness. This works like a painkiller, where fear and anger go away for a short moment but then come back when the meditation ends. With analytic meditation we can get to the root cause of the fear or the anger.
>
> Many people think meditation simply means sitting and closing your eyes. That kind of meditation even my cat can do. He sits there very calmly purring. If a rat comes by, he has nothing to worry about. We Tibetans often recite mantras so much like *Om Mani Padua Hum*, a mantra invoking the name of the Buddha of Compassion, that we forget to really investigate the root of our suffering. (Dalai Lama et al., 2016, pp. 315–316)

The Book of Joy (2016) suggests: "Pick a topic or experience that is troubling you, or simply watch your thoughts and feelings arise and recognize that they are temporary, without judging or identifying with them. . . . Now ask yourself, 'Is my thought true? How do I know for sure? Does it help the situation? Is there a better way of thinking about it or approaching the situation?'" (p. 317).

Wilson Hurley (2021), in his book *Compassion's Compass*, argues for using the kind of contemplation that fits the circumstance. That is, if your mind seems to be jumping all over the place and your nervous system is jangled, then the well-known technique of focusing on your breath may help. Hurley also advocates integrating some techniques from CBT, such as identifying cognitive distortions: "These passive and more active styles of working with one's mind are not seen as contradictory but as different approaches that can be used by a single person for different purposes" (p. 29).

Finally, your client may find one or more of the modern mindfulness apps to their liking. CALM includes a short, approximately seven-minute "daily calm" meditation. Some clients find that it gives them something to think about during the day, and, as it is short, they can fit it into their schedule. And Headspace, full of many different forms of meditation, is even available now on United Airline flights.

Many people pray. Unfortunately, early psychologists or psychiatrists were openly anti-religious, so it may surprise your client if you ask whether praying has helped in the past. However, asking may provide an opening to discuss other important questions, such as if they were raised in a religious family, what they have practiced in the past or are now practicing, how they find meaning in life, and how they believe their religion might be able to help to reduce their current distress.

Research (Captari et al., 2018; Captari et al., 2022) also suggests that for your religious clients, it will be very useful to discuss with them how their religious beliefs help them be more accepting. For Epictetus, the founder of Stoicism, everything was a manifestation of God's will. It made no sense to upset oneself over what was happening. The key was to accept. The second line of the Lord's Prayer, the most important prayer in Christianity, states, "Thy will be done."

One time I was working in Nigeria with a wonderful group of very devout Christian therapists and counselors. The government had suddenly raised the price of gasoline and the country was in turmoil. Everyone in the workshop had to drive home, and some lived far away from Abeokuta, where the workshop was being held. Many of them were very anxious about arriving home safely despite their Christian faith. The situation led to a deep conversation about the conflict between their strong religious beliefs and faith and their strong beliefs about the dangers and what might happen on their way home. It was important to everyone in the group to pray before they left.

In your client's religion, what would help them accept? Going to a temple or church and lighting a candle? Praying? Fasting? Going on a pilgrimage? When truly dreadful things happen in a client's life, no amount of therapy of any kind may be sufficient. Something older, with deeper roots in their lives, may be needed.

Risk-Taking Exercises

A good risk-taking exercise involves an activity in line with a client's goals and values but one that they might normally avoid. Perhaps an important email needs to be sent. Or perhaps a phone call to a difficult parent is long overdue. Or asking someone out on a date would be helpful. Neuroimaging research into the plasticity of the human brain has clearly demonstrated that we can "retrain" or "rewire" our brain when we do things that parts of our brain are reluctant to do.

I often give a risk-taking exercise to my students as a homework assignment. In one class, discussing what they had done, a young woman told the class that she had been working in a retail outlet for about three years. Her supervisor came to her and said, "We need to write up Nancy because she is really not working out, but I know you don't like to do that, so I'll do it for you." But the student said, "No. I'll do it," and she did. Later when she told the class about her experience, it was very evident that she was extremely pleased with her new behavior, one could say her new "self." She was no longer behaving like a shy, insecure teenager. She was pushing herself to stand up as an adult (she had just turned 21) and do what was necessary.

Another student reported that she avoided calling her mother because her mother was always critical. In line with her values, she thought she should call her at least once per week. For the class homework assignment, she did so, and survived! In fact, she said the conversation went better than she had expected and, again, it was very, very clear that she felt better about herself.

Clients who want very much to find another job but are avoiding sending out emails may be helped more by a homework assignment that helps them write and send three emails than any form of talk-only therapy. In addition, while discussing what type of homework assignment might be helpful, the therapist and the client gain further insight into the rigid, inflexible thinking that is getting in the client's way.

Help Clients Reduce Experiential Avoidance

Hayes's concept of "experiential avoidance" has great merit. It focuses on the *impact* of avoidance as a behavior. In 1955 and later, Ellis upset the psychoanalytic community with his revolutionary idea: It is not your mother. It is your own "low frustration tolerance (LFT)" that is often the problem. Then Linehan tweaked that to "low distress tolerance," a good tweak. Hayes's "experiential avoidance" correctly puts the focus on what we may do when faced with frustration or distress and how that may become reinforced and then repeated.

In *Get Out of Your Mind & Into Your Life,* Hayes (2005) points out that many people do not want to experience the discomfort that may arise, so they avoid doing something—perhaps something important—altogether. The wonderful video "Headstuck! What iIs Experiential Avoidance?" on YouTube (https://www.youtube.com/watch?v=C-ZuqeyxULM) is often a great help to clients and students.

There are many ways that you can help clients reduce experiential avoidance. "If-then" statements help people do what they intend to do when the time arrives. For example:

"If it is 4:00 p.m., I'll go to the gym."
"If I start feeling very anxious, I'll take some slow, deep breaths."
"If it is 10:00 p.m., I'll start getting ready for bed."
"If I'm about to have sex with X, I'll use a condom."

Many research studies into "implementation intentions" (Gollwitzer & Sheeran, 2006) have clearly shown that this type of planning and these types of statements increase the odds that someone who *intends* to do X will actually do X when the time or situation arises. For example, when some clients are alone, they may impulsively go on Tinder, even though they know, perhaps from experience, that hooking up with someone, especially a stranger, ultimately will make them feel worse. "If-then" statements can help. They can be almost like posthypnotic suggestions. Without thinking, instead of reaching for their phone, they can respond differently (e.g., call a friend, watch another episode of *Mrs. Maisel*, take a hot shower, and/or practice just sitting and observing the feeling of being lonely rather than obsessively looking to "fix" it).

You can also help your client come up with concrete, behavioral ways of moving toward their goals ("shaping" their behavior, to use Skinner's language) and decreasing experiential avoidance. Goals such as "study more," "get more As" or "be a better student" may sound good, but they are much too vague. There is no way to measure them during the week. They (and you) cannot tell if they are doing better until the end of the term, much too late. Help them use (1) time or (2) something like the number of words written or pages read to shape their behavior.

Like many people, your client may like the Pomodoro technique, which uses a timer to help people stay on task. They can set the timer and study for 20-, 30-, or 45-minute intervals. The "rules" include no answering the phone (even better, having it turned off), no checking emails, no watching YouTube clips, no cleaning up the kitchen—in fact, some people choose, no leaving the chair until the time is up. Just sitting may be very uncomfortable, but most people eventually find a way to work. They also often gain insight into the way perfectionism, discomfort, and experiential avoidance play a negative role in their lives.

Alternatively, if they are trying to write a paper, a different behavioral goal, number of words instead of number of minutes can help them get done what they want to *have done* later in the day, for example, to have written 200, 500, or 1,000 words, or whatever seems reasonable. When the number is reached, they should be encouraged to reward themselves, for example, with celebratory self-talk—"I did it! I did it!"—or something else that the two of you can determine. Rewards like watching a YouTube video "for only 20 minutes" may not work because they may have great difficulty stopping once they start.

Some people were born more antsy and more impulsive than others. It *is* more difficult for them to stay on task. Using behavioral techniques may help them learn to manage such an "antsy" nervous system better. At the same time, they may get done what they want to have gotten done, which almost always is therapeutic.

Take-Home Therapy Exercises

Given that we have only 45–50 minutes to work with our clients, having them do an ABC(DE) worksheet at home is a major time-saver. When someone takes home a form (and I always give two, so they don't feel that they have to be super-careful filling it in) or downloads it, fills it in, and then brings it back, we can quickly see what they are thinking and what they understand and don't understand. It is another example of how between-session work is very helpful in the ongoing assessment process.

You may have done a cost–benefit analysis (CBA; see chapter 14) in session, but a month later it may be good to ask a client to do another one, this time at home. It is an excellent way to enhance and maintain motivation.

Affirming Strengths: What Has Your Client Done Well or Is Proud Of?

Automatized, chronic, negative voices often consistently overwhelm positive ones. Some research suggests that that is the brain's default. When someone is not thinking of anything in particular, the brain is wired to scan the horizon for anything that might be amiss or left undone or needs to be done or dangerous or. . . . It is great for surviving, but, unfortunately,

**Textbox 8.1. Research Note #3: We Know What Works.
Why Don't We Do It?**

Not all children know how to be a student in school. However, if we help them
learn in the first grade how to "do" school, that is, how to be good students, 15
years later, they will be doing much, much better than those who just happen, by
luck (random assignment), to have been put in classrooms without the intervention. From classrooms with the program, only 29% of aggressive/disruptive first
graders were abusing or dependent on drugs 15 years later. From the classrooms
without the program, 83%. Zero percent of first graders who were lucky enough to
be assigned to the program smoked 10 or more cigarettes a day. Those not lucky
enough to be in the program, 40%.

Of those who later used school-based services for problems with behavior,
emotions, or drugs or alcohol, among the troubled first graders not in the program: 33%. Among similar boys who were in the program, only 17%.

How was this achieved? What was the intervention? No pills, just a simple
game—the Good Behavior Game—in first grade (Kellam et al., 2011). Nothing
after that. And the intervention took no time away from the regular school lessons.

In the schools with the program, students were divided into small groups. Children who had been identified by their teachers as especially aggressive or disruptive
were dispersed among the groups. The teacher explained how the game worked
and during the lesson would announce when it had begun. Groups of students who
maintained the announced behavior—sitting in their chair, doing their math problems, and so on—got stickers. Those who did not got check marks. Initially, the
game was run for only short periods of time (e.g., five to 10 minutes). Later it was
run for longer periods and, eventually, students were not even told when it began.

Why did it work? First, it assumed that not all students know how to be a student
in school and that some students need more help than others. The students in the
group helped each other learn and get stickers and avoid checks, especially those
who were having the most difficulty in their early days in school.

The program has been studied throughout the world and has demonstrated a
positive impact on later diagnosis of antisocial personality disorder and attention
deficit/hyperactivity, early onset of smoking, and peer rejection (Nolan et al.,
2014). Another study found a reduction in suicide attempts (Wilcox et al., 2008).
Given such dramatic results over time, it is difficult to understand why such a
program is not in all schools.

terrible for thriving. Consequently, many clients have to actively counteract those negative,
worrying voices.

Writing a list of things that they have done and are pleased with or proud of helps provide
balance. There are many lists that clients can make that may help them realize their potential,
including "10 Personal Characteristics That I Like about Myself" and "10 Things That I Enjoy
Doing." Printing a list and occasionally looking at it helps, too.

Textbox 8.2. Case—Ravi: Quieting a Storm

Ravi, a rising executive in a financial company, had had a panic attack on the subway. The EMS people had to come and carry him out on a stretcher. Then he had to go to the emergency room. It was, according to him, the most humiliating, terrifying experience that he had ever had. In his view, he absolutely could not stand having another attack, certainly not on the subway. So, he was completely avoiding subways and finding other ways to get around the city.

I knew the standard ABC technique to help uncover what Ravi was telling himself to make things even worse, for example, *I must not ever have an attack like that. I cannot stand going into the subway.* But I didn't think that would be helpful in the first session. Instead, we started to work together to uncover what might have contributed to his attack.

Ravi had been anxious most of his life. His mother is also a very anxious person, so I suggested that there was a genetic component. I told him about Jerome Kagan's study (see Research Note, chapter 13) and that Kagan had found that some very young babies were much more reactive than others. They grow up, I noted. Maybe Ravi had a very reactive nervous system.

I asked him if he drank coffee, and he said yes.

"Eight cups a day?" I asked with a big smile. I was using a technique I learned when I was in training. Exaggerate—with a big smile. Make it sound really outlandish, and you will probably get something closer to the truth.

"What? Are you crazy?" he answered, also with a smile.

"Well, I don't know. How much?"

"I have two big Starbucks in the morning."

"So that could have contributed to the attack," I said. "Was there anything else going on that day? You mentioned earlier that you were having problems with your girlfriend."

"Yes. I feel really trapped in this relationship, but I don't know what I'm going to do."

"And are you still worried about work?"

"Yes. They're laying off a lot of people, and I may be next."

"And are you still going to the gym?"

"No. I just don't have time with what is going on at the office."

"That sounds like a perfect storm."

"What do you mean?"

I wanted him to stop blaming himself for what had happened, which he was doing: *It was so stupid. I don't know what happened.* I suggested that there were five factors that combined and led to him having a panic attack: Genetic/underlying anxiety; a lot of coffee; feeling trapped in a relationship; being afraid that he was about to lose his job; no exercising.

"I don't think your body liked that combination. So, it went a bit berserk, and you wound up on the subway platform," I added.

He looked confused.

"Weather people say that four factors must come together to produce a tornado. Missing one of those, no tornado. For you, five factors came together, and your body had had enough. Which of those factors could you eliminate? Ask the girl-friend to leave?" I said with a smile.

He sat for a while. "No, I'm not ready to do that. Near, but not yet. Cut down the caffeine, I guess."

"That would help. You can't change your genes, but you can reduce the amount of caffeine. That would make your nervous system less reactive and more resilient. And exercise would help, too. Could you get some exercise?"

"I have a gym membership. I just haven't been going."

"What could you do to get at least some exercise?"

"I could walk to work."

"That sounds like a great idea. A doable idea. If you do nothing, a new tornado may occur. And, of course, you can make everything worse by telling yourself stuff like, *I can't stand it if another attack occurs on the subway*," I said, with a smile.

"What do you mean?"

"Well, telling yourself, *This must not happen. I can't stand it if it happens again* will add a sixth factor, a vicious-cycle feedback loop. At the slightest twinge of anxiety, you're going to tighten up and you'll start to get even more anxious. If you said to yourself instead, 'I really don't want this to happen, but if it does, it isn't the end of the world,' it wouldn't be as likely to happen. If you're not careful, you are going to have what we call a secondary problem, panic about panic. You don't need any more problems!"

Then I shifted gears. "Why did you think it was so humiliating?"

"I was lying there on the ground. People were gathered around staring at me. I had to be carried out."

"What do you think the people were thinking?"

"I don't know. 'Look at him. What a jerk? I'm so glad I'm not there.'"

"So, if I have a heart attack, and fall on the ground and everyone is staring at me, that is what I'm supposed to think and feel? Humiliation, and that the people staring at me are thinking, 'Oh, my god. What a jerk!'"

"No. But a heart attack is different!"

"How so? Maybe I contributed to mine by eating too much fat and not taking any medication, and you contributed to yours by drinking too much coffee. I'm not stressed out about losing my job, but you are. What's the difference?"

He sat there. "I don't know," he said.

"It's up to you. You can feel humiliated and never get on a subway again, or you can think about it differently. By the way, someone in the crowd might have been thinking, 'What a loser!' Do you really care what someone who thinks like that thinks? You are a more compassionate person than that. I don't know you very well, but I know that. Why don't you give yourself a little self-compassion. And cut out some of the coffee, too.

"Returning to our original question, what can you do this week to greatly reduce the likelihood of a tornado, that is, a panic attack, which I know is a very, very disagreeable experience? Not the end of the world, but extremely, extremely dis-agreeable. What can you do?"

"I guess I can drink less coffee."

"Yes, buy one. Or buy half-caff. Ask them to fill it half with caffeinated coffee and half with decaf. What else?"

"I could walk to work."

"Yes. Exercise is the cheapest antidepressant, antianxiety, anti-panic attack 'medicine' that you can take. It works wonders. And?"

He looked confused.

"As long as you keep thinking 'I absolutely *must never* have a panic attack, especially in the subway again,' you'll be more prone to have one. I didn't say you *will* have one, but you'll be more prone to have one. You need to change the way you think about passing out and being on your back on the subway platform. When you come back next week, I'll give you an exercise to help you with that. But do you think you could take a short trip when it is not so crowded, perhaps with a friend?"

"Yes. Maybe."

"Well, that would help. But without cutting down on the caffeine and getting some exercise, that may not work, okay?"

"Yes."

The following week, I remembered to check on his homework at the beginning of the next session. He had walked to work, was drinking only one large Starbucks in the morning, and had gone on the subway with his friend to a party.

"And you didn't die. Fantastic," I said, with a big smile.

Sleep, Wearables, and Smartphones

As I have noted before, many clients—and clinicians—are sold on the idea that if they just understand the roots of their problems, they will feel and do better. It is difficult for them to accept the critical role of changing behaviors in addition to gaining insight. If people don't get enough sleep, they'll feel more anxious and depressed, they'll have more difficulty managing their anger, and they'll get less done and do it less well. The research is completely clear about that (Krizan & Hisler, 2019; Pandi-Perumal et al., 2020; Rosa et al., 1983).

How much sleep does your client need on average to function well? Many clients don't know. To become more aware about their sleep, they can purchase a wearable like a Fitbit or use their smartphone. This is a good between-session assignment. Knowing how much sleep, on average, they need often contributes significantly to doing and feeling better overall.

People are very resistant to changing their sleep habits even though they complain about often being tired. They don't want to bother to lie down on a mattress for six or eight or perhaps even more hours. Who has the time? As a result, many people have trained themselves to get by on less sleep than they actually need. It may be very difficult for you to convince them that more sleep might help them as much as therapy. Many people also do not know or believe that some people need nine hours of sleep to be healthy; a few even need 10.5 hours. No doubt, it is very difficult for such people to fit into modern society. It is a genuine burden, of a sort. However, not acknowledging the reality that genetics has given them will certainly add to the harm the lack of sufficient sleep can do.

Your client may have been brainwashed by our culture. They simply do not have enough time in a day to sleep more. And, unfortunately for them, some of their friends can get by with much less sleep. Thomas Edison reportedly slept about four hours a night and was perhaps more responsible than anyone else for initiating the productivity culture. In his mind, more productive people are better people and sleeping is not productive. Fortunately, the research that shows that the lack of sleep contributes to an increased likelihood of dying of cancer and heart disease is gradually causing people to take the importance of sleep more seriously.

In some cases, clients should be encouraged to see a psychopharmacologist or go to a sleep lab. Getting too little sleep night after night can lead to a psychotic break. Getting too much sleep contributes to depression. Finding the balance between awfulizing and being appropriately concerned is not easy. Although over the long run a non-medication solution may be found, preventing a psychotic break is more important. Medications may be needed.

Exercise, Wearables, and Smartphones

Exercise is the least expensive antidepressant, antianxiety "medication" available. If I can get a client back to some form of exercising, that almost always helps them feel and do better. Again, Fitbits, other wearables, and smartphone apps can play a very motivating and health-promoting role.

ACT's "Attending Your Own Funeral" Exercise

ACT's "Attending Your Own Funeral" exercise (see p. 166 in *Get Out of Your Mind & Into Your Life* [2015]) is a powerful, motivating exercise designed to move people to take action, guided by their values and, ultimately, to do more of what they want to have done with their lives. According to the directions, you (assuming you are doing this exercise) are first asked to write down what you are afraid might be said at your funeral if you "back off from what you really want to stand for, and instead you follow a path of avoidance, mental entanglement, emotional control, and self-righteousness" (p. 167). Then you are asked to write what you fear someone might be thinking inside their head but not saying. Finally, you are asked to write what you would like to be in a eulogy about you: "Let these words reflect the meaning you would most like to create, the purposes you would most like to reveal about the time you spent on this planet" (p. 167).

Chapter 9

Working with Diverse Clients

Before moving on to the next section of the book, it is important to acknowledge that if we counselors and psychotherapists are going to make a true effort to work with more diverse clients, we need to listen to how they frame their distress and learn from other ways of healing. If we signal that our evidence-based methods are superior to traditional customs and healing methods, Ethan Watters, in *Crazy Like Us: The Globalization of the American Psyche* (2010), suggests that we are perpetuating an attitude very similar to those held by the colonizing people of the past three centuries. Unfortunately, American thinking often seems to be that if people have psychological or behavioral difficulties, they should take a pill or work on their thinking or do both. That tends to ignore other factors that may be contributing to their problems.

The research is now clear: Poverty leads to more adverse childhood events (ACEs; Felitti et al, 1998; Felitti et al., 2019) and more ACEs lead to more health problems in adult life (see chapter 2, p. 13). Ellis and Dietz (2017) have added adverse community environments to the original ACE model (i.e., poverty, discrimination, poor housing quality and availability, community violence, and lack of opportunity, economic mobility, and social capital).

How much one earns is often equated in clients' minds with how "good" or "worthless failures" they are. In fact, clients are much more uncomfortable talking about how much they earn than sex, or practically anything else. During the summer, some children go to a YMCA camp, but others go to very expensive private camps. Who they meet, mingle and play with will be significantly different. In the latter case, if they are scholarship campers or from families that could barely pay the fees, they may feel marginalized and humiliated. Several driven, overworking clients of mine have grappled all their lives to overcome the impact of slights and humiliations from their childhood camp experiences.

Race, as a concept, was invented for political purposes. It helped powerful groups assert their right to privileges and wealth and deny them to other groups. Considering that it continues to be used for such purposes, it matters. Redlining and other techniques were used by banks for decades, starting before the Civil War, to prevent people of color from purchasing property, especially homes. Consequently, their children did not inherit the accumulated wealth that has accrued to many white families over the years. Without accrued wealth, it continues to be more difficult to get mortgages and buy homes. Two huge housing developments in New York City, Stuyvesant Town and Peter Cooper Village, were built by the Metropolitan Insurance Company after WWII with help from New York City, but "negroes" were not allowed to apply or live there. Separate buildings were constructed for them in Harlem.

What does this have to do with counseling and psychotherapy? Most New Yorkers do not know that apartheid was practiced in New York City less than 100 years ago. But many African Americans in New York City do know. Moreover, as noted above, research now clearly shows that poverty affects psychological and physical development. Western psychology has been developed primarily by white men from privileged backgrounds. Historically, white researchers, mostly men, have used participants from various racial groups without their permission, sometimes in heinous ways, for example, at the Tuskegee Institute. This, too, may have an impact on your working alliance with some clients.

Most researchers were also devoted to developing a science of psychotherapy and did not include the study of religious beliefs or practices. As noted earlier, most early psychotherapists and counselors were secular in their approach and even, at times, explicitly anti-religious. However, most of my clients are religious. They are often serious about trying to live a life in line with their religious beliefs, that is, to be a good Jew, Christian, Muslim, Sikh, Hindu, and so on. Moreover, CBT theory asserts that a client's beliefs have a major impact on how we feel and act. What about a client's beliefs about God or gods and His/Her/Their role in your client's life? No doubt, a client's religious and spiritual beliefs may have a major influence on the way they experience anxiety and depression and the way they think and feel about their behavior.

In one sense, the Buddha was the first "cognitive behavior" therapist. He asserted that everyone will suffer in life, but one can make things better or worse by how one processes that suffering. The gods (or devils) are not the cause. What matters is how we respond to what is happening. The Eightfold Path, including Right Thinking and Right Action, was the answer.

For centuries, people in the West have, in fact, had a drive or desire "to become someone." In contrast, in the East, the focus has been on spiritual growth and on the community. Edward Conze (1959) in *Buddhism: Its Essence and Development*, notes, "The indigenous tradition of Europe is inclined to affirm the will to live, and to turn actively towards the world of the senses. The spiritual tradition of mankind is based on the negation of the will to live and is turned away from the world of the senses. All European spirituality has had to be periodically renewed by an influx from the East" (p. 12). The introduction of mindfulness to counseling and therapy is the most recent example.

Your clients' distress may also be caused by the fact that in many regions and families, members of their nuclear family, their extended family, and their churches or temples may completely disown them. Fortunately, in many parts of the United States, it is far easier now for young people to acknowledge that they may be homosexual or bisexual or a bit of both, "fluid," and to break from the norms of their culture and religion. But given the quickly changing legal landscape in some states and in various countries abroad, many clients are experiencing significant levels of stress, anxiety, and depression. Your client may also be uncomfortable being a first-time-to-college student at an Ivy League university, a non-white student at the same institution, transgender, or all three.

Finally, in the intense discussions about diversity, equity, and inclusion during the past decade, physical and psychological disabilities have often been neglected. The Americans with Disabilities Act is more than 30 years old, and companies and cities have made efforts to be more accommodating to people with disabilities, but many barriers remain. The legal ADA requirements may be met, but little thought or attention given to the actual accommodations. Space is made for wheelchairs at concert halls, but often they are in the front row on the side or in the very back row. Even though there are over a billion people with disabilities on the planet, representing a market larger than the United States, Brazil, Pakistan, and Indonesia combined, the cost of a vehicle capable of taking a wheelchair is still beyond the reach of most people.

One study (Narayanan & Terris, 2020) found that productivity was greater among factory teams with a higher proportion of people with disabilities compared to the productivity of teams with a lower proportion, but employment opportunities remain limited. However, if people with serious psychological difficulties such as a bipolar disorder or major depression opt to go on Social Security Disability Income and then decide they would feel and be better if they worked, they can risk the loss of their benefits for six months or more, including their access to necessary medications. As a result, they are caught in a catch-22 situation where they wish to enhance their life with a job but are appropriately anxious about the consequences of doing so.

WHAT CAN YOU DO?

Practice Humility

Multicultural counseling (Hilert & Tirado, 2019; Ridley et al., 1994; Ridley et al., 2021) has been the focus of considerable work and controversy (Helms, 1994; Mollen & Ridley, 2021; Vandiver et al., 2021) for the past 30 years, and working with people from different cultures and classes can be very challenging. It is particularly challenging given how diverse cultures are, as well. In New York City alone, each neighborhood (e.g., Astoria, Williamsburg, Harlem, the Upper West Side, and the Upper East Side) has its own culture and within each neighborhood, each family has its own microculture. In biracial and bicultural families, ways of thinking and goals and values may have conflicted in significant ways for your client and, possibly, still conflict.

According to the US government, people from the Dominican Republic, Puerto Rico, Cuba, and Mexico are all simply "Hispanic," but when other factors such as class and skin color get factored in, the situation becomes much more complicated. My Trinidadian friend does not like being lumped with either "Black," "African American," or "West Indian," but multicultural researchers who are trying to expand their pool of participants invariably do so. As clinicians, how can we respond?

Hook (2014; Hook & Davis, 2019; Hook et al. 2016) has suggested that practicing humility may be better than taking courses in multicultural counseling, although doing both might be the best course of action. Humility in a counselor appears to be positively related to better working alliances and therapy outcomes. As we are so accustomed to doing when a client is describing their experience of depression or with trauma, we can listen and try to not let our unconscious biases interfere with our work.

Zhang and colleagues (2022) have defined cultural humility as "a way of being that involves a willingness, an openness and a desire to (a) reflect on *oneself* as an embedded cultural being and (b) hear about and strive to understand others' cultural backgrounds and identities" (p. 553). Their review of 21 studies of the impact of cultural humility on psychotherapy found that it was related to better outcomes (e.g., a more positive working alliance and more therapy continuance). It was also related to fewer and less impactful racial microaggressions.

Acting as if you understand just because you have known someone closely or think you have had similar experiences in life is probably an erroneous assumption. It is better to assume that you do not understand. People are so different and their experiences in society growing up so different that it is better to be curious and ask questions.

Self-Reflection and Meditation

Some form of brief or extended meditation may help. As mentioned in the previous chapter, there are many, quite different forms of meditation. Taking time to quietly sit and observe one's thinking about the various issues discussed in this chapter will help you become more aware of your own biases and blind spots. Doing so will help you become a more effective clinician (Burgess et al., 2017; Hilert & Tirado, 2019; Wong & Vinsky, 2021). You do not have to sit for

30 minutes. Many people do not feel they can take 30 minutes. Sitting for five minutes will help. Five minutes is also better than no minutes at all.

Do No Harm

As you know, a physician's most important rule is Do No Harm. Ample evidence exists that significant disparities in health care exist in the United States, including cancer treatment (dos-Santos-Silva et al., 2022), emergency room visits (Soares et al., 2019), and amputations (Stapleton et al., 2018). When professionals refuse to or simply do not look at their own unconscious biases (Marcelin et al., 2019) and how those biases may affect their thinking and the care they provide, they may do harm (Arora et al., 2022).

As counselors and psychotherapists, what can you do to avoid perpetuating this situation? Despite the fact that it may cause discomfort, undercovering our underlying biases and noticing how they may affect our thinking and behavior is crucial to becoming a better clinician. As Fitzgerald (2000) writes, "It is about developing the ability to 'see' a situation from multiple perspectives and, if necessary, to reconcile them. It is about developing multiple potential interpretations and using critical reflective thinking to choose which alternatives are most likely to provide effective strategies for care. It is about using such understandings to become more competent and effective professionals" (pp. 184–185).

Do No Self-Blaming

What is key is that we do not think to ourselves, "I shouldn't think that way" and/or "They shouldn't think that way." The result may be defensiveness and anger and may block further insight and growth. You were raised in a culture with its beliefs and stereotypes. That is inescapable. As you are working together, why not ask questions like, "Am I missing something?" "Is there something that if I could get in your shoes I would think differently about?" "Is there something about the culture where you are living or where you come from that may affect this problem?"

Fortunately, millions of people in the United States are committed to being more accepting of people who are different from them, trying to understand what it is like to be in an ethnic minority or to be transgender or to be non-white. Many of the students I taught at the College at Old Westbury specifically went there because it was the most diverse college in the SUNY system, and they wanted to get to know and make friends with people from different cultural and ethnic groups.

Be Mindful of Microaggressions

Much has been written about microaggressions over the past 10 years (see especially Sue et al., 2007), and for a bit of amusement, see https://www.youtube.com/watch?v=DWynJkN5HbQ. The whole concept is annoying to some, often white, often male people. "Why are some people so sensitive?" they ask. But often they have never been the subject of microaggressions. Again, we now know that repeated stressors over time are harmful to people not only psychologically but also physically. (See the ACE studies, and studies into the impact of trauma on the hippocampus, Woon et al., 2010.)

The research (see below) by Hook and his associates (2016) suggests that asking clients about possible microaggressions that may have occurred during therapy may help. The more aware or mindful a counselor can become of the way they may inadvertently step on other people's toes, the more likely they will be effective with diverse clients.

Use Motivational Interviewing

Open-ended questions and Rogerian-style active listening work well. There is no reason that you should know everything when it comes to someone else's culture or sexual orientation or psychological or physical problems. Building on the skills that you learned from school and workshops, you can develop more effective ways to work with diverse clients, provided that you remain curious and open to learning. Using your MI skills—and practicing them—will move you along to becoming a more expert practitioner with a diverse population of clients.

Textbox 9.1. Research Note #4: Microaggressions and Therapy

Hook and colleagues (2016), in a fairly large-scale study (n = 2212) of a reasonably diverse group (30.9% Hispanic, 29.7% Black, 12.4%, Asian, 6% American Indian, 17.5% multiracial), reported that microaggressions were infrequently felt in therapy (1.77 on a 1–5 scale where 1 = never and 5 = always). However, more than 80% reported experiencing at least one. The most common seemed to be counselors avoiding or denying the impact of culture or acting as if it didn't exist. At a minimum, counselors were uncomfortable talking about it.

Interestingly, microaggressions were more often reported when the client and counselor were matched in terms of ethnicity. Perhaps clients expect more of a counselor who comes from the same ethnic background. Alternatively, perhaps class differences played a role in such situations, a factor that was not explored.

Help Clients Accept Their Neurodivergence

The concept of "normal" originally came from mathematics. A perpendicular angle was defined as "normal." It was also seen by some mathematicians as a reflection of the divine and therefore somehow "right." A 90-degree angle became known as a "right angle," even though there is nothing right or left about it. Very unfortunately, the idea of "normal" became somehow "right" and "good," and that stuck. Hence, being abnormal is inherently less than good.

Early psychiatrists focused on illnesses and that also got tied in with "abnormal" and with the *DSM* "disorders." Today, if your client wants counseling or therapy and wants to get reimbursed by an insurance company, they have to go along with some kind of "disorder" attached to their name.

Some people are beginning to push back against such a medicalization of what they see as a different nervous system, not "disordered," and not better or worse. They see themselves as "neurodivergent." This way of looking at the way their nervous system functions has at least two advantages. First, they stop blaming and shaming themselves for behaviors that they now understand from a different vantage point. Other people may have labeled them as "stupid," "self-centered," and "lazy," and they may have been criticized or made fun of because of their difficulties. Partly as the result of not understanding their differences, they may have flunked out of two or three colleges and have shifted jobs—or lost jobs—many times. Being kinder to themselves and accepting that they did not choose to have these problems is a key first step in feeling better about themselves and often doing better, as well.

Textbox 9.2. Case—Joanna and the Role of Her Faith

One client, Joanna, a devout Christian, and I were almost finished with the session when she said, "I still really think that I should be able to have a better relationship with my husband. When he gets drunk, which is not that often but often enough, he is nasty to the children. He doesn't hit them or yell at them, but he is snide and critical and says he is ashamed of them. I really hate that."
"How can your religion help with this?" I asked.

Joanna and I had been talking about many difficult problems in her life. She had married young and had always tried to live a very principled life. Her husband had had a drinking problem throughout their 10-year marriage, but, she said, he had been a very good man in many ways. He had built a successful company, had treated his employees fairly, and was kind and loving to her, except when he was drinking.

Joanna and I went on to talk about the second story in the Bible. It grapples with who is responsible for one's actions. Although the Adam and Eve story can be interrupted as a story about sex and guilt and the consequences that flow from not obeying, one can also see it as a "passing the buck" story. Neither Adam nor Eve will take responsibility for their actions.

What was her responsibility at this point in her life, in her marriage, and in the life of her children? What was God's?

I asked her about how she interpreted the line in the Lord's Prayer, "Thy will be done." In her mind, that did not necessarily mean that only God's will exists. According to her, if it is God's will for you or me to become the best therapist or mother or lawyer or chef that we can be, then it is our job to work on ourselves so that we can blossom in the way God wished for us.

Earlier in the session, I had pointed out that she was and is a very principled person and that several important principles were in conflict. She had vowed to stay with her husband "through sickness and health." At the same time, she also believed two other important principles: (1) A mother should always do what she can to protect her children, and (2) a husband should not speak to his wife or children in an abusive manner.

I asked her what she thought she could do in the coming week to help her with this conflict. She was quite clear: She should pray every night. Two times in her past, going to her church and lighting a candle had had an enormous impact. Because I thought it might help her move forward, I suggested she do the same thing this time, and she agreed. I knew it would take time for her to resolve the conflict. For her, lighting a candle might help her sustain hope and give her the courage to take whatever actions she decided to take.

Such conversations are common in my office. Anxiety, depression, addictions, and so forth are all affected by what we think is our place in a larger context. Our client's ideas about the role of God, gods, fate, or genes in their life can have a profound impact on how helpful therapy is. Ignoring religious and spiritual beliefs is as bad as ignoring the role of neurochemistry, exercise, or sleep.

Second, they can begin to focus on how to better manage and take advantage of the nervous system that they have. They can see their nervous system as divergent but not abnormal or disordered. In fact, your client may be more creative than other people or they may be able to see a problem from a different angle that is beneficial to an entire project.

"Consultation" versus "Therapy"

For some clients, having therapy and counseling covered by health insurance like any other illness was a big step forward. But other clients may prefer to see their problem as just that, a problem, not an illness. If they have a tax problem, they consult with a tax accountant. If they have stomach pain, they consult an internist. Considering that mental illness is still seen as something to be ashamed of and hidden by most people in most cultures, framing a session as a "consultation," perhaps only one, may help increase the appeal of counseling and therapy. Hall and colleagues (2021), for example, suggest that when helping Asian clients, "pragmatic intervention approaches focused on helping individuals cope with specific external problems, compared to managing a 'personal' disease, can effectively 'restore' face. Thus, social problem-solving interventions may be more personally relevant to many people of East Asian ancestry than are approaches that are internally focused" (p. 91).

Watch Foreign Films

If you cannot or do not live in a multicultural city and you do not have the resources or inclination to travel, watching foreign films can be immensely helpful. No doubt, foreign films are often made by people who grew up in the middle or upper middle class of their society, but the clients you see may come from a similar class.

Of course, foreign films are more difficult to watch than films from the culture you are familiar with. In addition, you may have to teach yourself how to read subtitles. But they allow you to enter a different world. In doing so, you may not only better understand some of your clients, but you may gain insight into your own personal struggles. Seeing that others struggle in similar ways in different cultures may help you accept your own difficulties. Seeing that others surmount their difficulties may also lift your own spirits.

PART III

Subsequent Sessions

Chapter 10

Ongoing Assessment, Evaluating Between-Session Work, Checking on Therapeutic Goals, and Setting the Agenda

In subsequent sessions, clients often start by bringing up something from the past week. This may be very relevant, but it may actually distract them from focusing on their true goals for therapy. Traditional therapy relies on talking to generate insight and on insight to resolve a client's problems. Clients often believe in the effectiveness of that approach, too. But insight may not be sufficient. Moreover, their therapeutic goals may get lost in the weekly ups and downs of their lives. The first parts of subsequent sessions present us with many opportunities to prevent this from happening.

WHAT CAN YOU DO?

Note: The following are not in any particular order. If you are not clear about the client's goals, you might start there and not with finding out about their between-session work. In the first part of any session, as was discussed in chapter 3, you should focus on building the working relationship.

Build the Relationship in Subsequent Sessions

Reread your notes before the session. Reflect upon whether you know what your client's goals are for therapy. Think about how you are going to evaluate between-session experiences (see below); that is one of the trickiest parts of any session. Learning how to do that without causing a client to feel judged is a critically important skill to develop.

You may also want to ask yourself, "What do *I* think we ought to work on?" Jot down in your notes or on the computer two to three things that you think you could work on if the client comes in with "nothing" to work on. Of course, when you make a suggestion, it is either going to be picked up by the client or not. In either case, you will probably learn something. Having your own thoughts on how you might proceed is not harmful unless you start to push your own agenda instead of listening for guidance from your client.

Session Outcome Assessment

Some clinicians make it part of their way of working to ask at the end of each session, "What was most meaningful to you about this session?" At the beginning of the second session and sometimes in subsequent sessions, I ask, "Was there anything I said when we met last time that was helpful and was there anything I said that was irritating?" This usually elicits information that is helpful for me in assessing not only the client but how they may have experienced the session. Remember that the nonverbal responses may be more important than the verbal ones.

There are a number of measures of the working alliance and of therapy outcomes that you may want to investigate, such as the Outcome Questionnaire 45 (OQ-45), Rating of Outcome Scale (ROS), Outcome Rating Scale (ORS), and the Psychological Outcomes Profiles Questionnaire (PSYCHLOPS). The latter is based on a radically different form of psychological measurement. Instead of giving the client a standard assessment instrument based on studying many clients, the client writes down on a form what they would like to monitor session to session. You can learn more about it at http://www.psychlops.org.uk/publications-and-studies.

Explore the Between-Session Experience

Evaluating between-session experiences is definitely a more challenging part of a session. Maybe that is why so many therapists avoid including between-session work in their therapy, or if they do suggest that a client do something, they forget to ask about it in the next session. Checking on between-session work will call on all of your motivational interviewing (MI) skills and more. If you have never studied MI, I suggest that you put that high on your to-do list. In this part of the session, the main risk is sounding like a parent or schoolteacher.

Several possibilities exist. Your client may have . . .

1. forgotten the agreed-upon, between-session work/homework altogether;
2. tried to do it but failed every time;
3. tried to do it but failed most of the time;
4. did it but succeeded only sometimes or only partially; or
5. completed it successfully.

Scenario #1: They Forgot

What does it mean if someone forgot to do the homework? This is surely an opportunity to learn more about your client. However, perhaps, first, it would be helpful to check your own emotional response. If you are disappointed, what are you telling yourself and how will your client respond to your disappointment? If you feel annoyed or irritated, what are you thinking? What does it mean to you? Later, after the session, should you speak to your supervisor? How would you like it if your therapist or supervisor showed that they were disappointed in you or annoyed?

Even feeling disappointed may be useful. It almost always means that you have become too invested in your client's progress. We are not coaches, although we may engage in some forms of coaching as a part of therapy (see chapter 18). Coaches frequently become very invested in their coachee's successes or failures. But that is not a good stance for therapists and counselors to take. If you become invested, you will probably find it impossible to be accepting and nonjudgmental of what your client tells you. Worse, your client may avoid telling you when things are going badly because they don't want to disappoint you or irritate you. That is, they start taking care of your emotional health!

For a long time, I have practiced what I call Zen caring. It is unrealistic not to care at all about how well or not well a client is doing. But if they forget to do their between-session work, what can we feel that will not injure the working relationship? We can feel genuinely curious. What happened? Why did it happen (forgetting or not doing the homework)? What does it mean? And we can feel grateful. It gives us an opportunity to learn something more about our client, maybe something very useful.

Let's assume that you are curious, open to learning, interested in better understanding your client. What can you say?

"Did you do your homework?" is clearly going to make you sound like their parent or fifth-grade teacher. As I discussed in chapter 4, trainers who teach MI encourage clinicians not to ask yes/no, closed-ended questions. When you do that, people feel interrogated. Even "Why didn't you do it?"—not a closed-end question—will probably be off-putting to most clients.

"How did things go this past week with what you were trying to do differently?" is a much better way to begin, with a curious, nonjudgmental tone and expression.

You may get the answer, "Oh, I forgot."

The way you respond is probably more an art than a science, although the research clearly indicates that confrontive or non-empathetic therapists do poorly and may even do harm (Moyers & Miller, 2013).

"Hmm, maybe it wasn't the right idea," may get some information.

To that, you might get, "No. I liked the idea. I meant to do it over the weekend, but I only remembered it when I was coming here."

Most traditional therapists do not include between-session work as part of therapy. Consequently, most clients aren't used to such an approach. It may take clients time to get into the habit of doing work between sessions.

Whether or not a client does anything will also probably be partly up to you. If you clearly signal that you think it is important, then they will probably do it more often. Dr. David Burns, the author of one of the best self-help books ever written, *Feeling Good* (2000), reportedly won't see clients who don't do homework. His research suggests that those who don't do homework don't get better, so doing therapy without homework seems unethical to him.

I understand his point and, of course, believe in behaving ethically. On the other hand, internists have lots of patients who don't regularly follow their advice, and they don't refuse to see them. In general, but not always, I follow that model. Something may change, and the client may start to do work between sessions or homework may simply not be helpful. But my experience shows, and the research indicates (Dobson, 2021) clearly, that clients do better when they do something between sessions, and I share that with my clients.

Scenarios #2 and #3: They Tried but Failed Every Time or Most of the Time

Your client intended to speak to their boss about a raise but didn't. Or they intended to call each of their siblings about something important, but only called two of the four. They tried to work on their dissertation and got nothing accomplished. They decided to ride the subway but couldn't get themselves to do it.

Again, whatever happens gives us and them an opportunity to learn. Many people who have "failed" in trying to do something become much more serious about therapy than they were before (see Caroline's case). Initial failure may be motivating not just discouraging. That depends a lot on how it gets processed.

However, maybe the assignment does need to be adjusted. While failing may help people move from one stage to another, too much failing is not going to be effective. What can you and they do to make success more likely? Change is very, very difficult if it terrifies your client. Change is also very, very difficult if it means changing a very automatized behavior and one that the brain misprocesses. But with a combination of tactics, you can help your client change.

Scenario #4: Partial Successes

Even those who successfully do some or all of their homework may do what CBT-ers call "discounting." I sometimes call it "but-ing": "I did it, but I only did some of it." "I did it, but I only did it once." "I did it, but I waited until the last moment." "I did it, but I should have done it a long time ago. What's wrong with me?" They find a hundred ways to discount their accomplishment.

If they did it some of the time but not all of the time, that gives you a wonderful opportunity to remind them that they are trying to learn *how* to do something differently. No one learns a new skill overnight—for example, how to hit a golf ball differently or how to get started on their work instead of YouTubing in the morning. Sometimes they will get it right and other times they won't. You need to reinforce that idea.

Scenario #5: Success

Skinner and other behaviorists say that you should definitely reinforce or reward a person who does the task they set out to do. And some therapists are very quick to say something congratulatory or encouraging. That may be fine, but it can lead to a client becoming dependent upon their therapist for positive feedback and reinforcement. It is much better that the clients themselves feel positive about what they have achieved. Therefore, you may want to take a little time making sure that they are savoring their accomplishment and not discounting. Many people who come to therapy are terrible about feeling positive when they have succeeded in doing something. It even makes some people anxious; in their past, good times were often followed by horrible times. As a result, they continue to be on guard, hypervigilant, very hesitant to savor what they have accomplished. This becomes another good goal for therapy. Savoring and enjoying when things go well.

Check on the Goals

Before or after checking on how the between-session work went, it is a good idea to check to make sure that you understand what the client wants to accomplish in therapy. Do you know their goals? As I have pointed out before, most modern therapy and counseling is future oriented and goal focused. You cannot very sensibly agree on an agenda for the session without knowing what you are trying to accomplish in the medium and long run.

A Rogerian approach may work best. Client-centered therapists often reflect to the client what they think the client has said: "If I get you right, an awful lot is going on at home. Your kids are home, and you have to help them with their schooling, your husband is too ill to help, you have your own job to do, and, of course, someone has to cook and clean, and that all falls on you. too. Do I have that right?"

"Yes."

"And you are here because you want to feel less depressed and less anxious, and you want to stop gaining weight, is that correct?"

"Yes."

"So, what would you like to work on first?"

Textbox 10.1. Case—Veronica: Too Busy and Exhausted to Do Anything Between Sessions, But . . .

Veronica, a young mother of three children and a working mom, had had a very difficult week. Her children were home because of COVID, and she and her husband had to work from home, too. Her husband had been bedridden with some kind of intestinal problem, not COVID related, for about a week, and everything had fallen on her shoulders. She had a chronic tendency to criticize herself and to worry about what she might not get done or what might happen. I had suggested that she might make a list of 10 things that she had done well in her life, and we had agreed upon that. Given what was going on in her house, I was pleased that she had not canceled the appointment, as she had the week before, but how could I ask her about my suggestion? I knew it was important, but I also thought she had probably not done it.

"How did it go with a list of things you have done well?" I asked. "Was it possible for you get that done with everything else going on?"

"No," she said. "I thought about it, but I just didn't have time."

"That's makes sense. It sounds like you have had almost a perfect storm at home this past week," I said. "And we definitely don't want to add one thing more for you to beat yourself up about."

We then talked about some issues in her childhood. Her mom had passed away when she was 17, and she had cared for her younger brother and sister, not only in the morning, getting them ready for school, but also in the evening. Before her mother died, she had worked two jobs to keep the family financially afloat. One hypothesis that we had was that she had two beliefs or "rules" in her head almost all the time: "You must work very hard or something very bad may happen." "Relaxing is for other people."

After we had talked about that for a while, I shifted gears. "Why don't we make the list right now? Would that be all right with you? No more 'problem talk' for a while. Tell me something you did between five and twenty that you are proud of?"

"I helped raise my brother and sister. But I also won the spelling bee in sixth grade. I was so proud."

She then rattled off three more accomplishments. After 10 minutes, we had a list of 11 accomplishments that she was proud of, four from ages 5 to 20, four from 20 to 30, and three from 30 until 35, her age at that point.

At the end of the session, she said, "Thank you for doing that. That was really helpful."

Set the Agenda

There is no "best way" to set the agenda. It depends mostly on the client but also on what you have in mind, as well. The question, "So what would you like to work on?" is a good way to start a session. Clients will often give you two or three things that they want to work on. Write them down, and then, during the session, try to ensure that you work on each. Of course, all of the time may be used on one item. In that case, you can note that that has happened and tell the client that you will work on the other items in the next session. Then, of course, it is important to do so. In addition, you may have noticed that at or near the end of a session, clients bring up something that they want to work on but have not brought up before. You can add this to the list.

When a client starts by talking about what happened during the past week, during a pause, I may ask, "OK, but what would you like to work on today?" or "Okay, that sounds very difficult. Is that what you would like to work on today or are there other things?"

Chapter 11

Facilitating Acceptance, Compassion, and Change: Mindfulness and Metastability

Hard to restrain, unstable is this mind; it flits wherever it lists. Good it is to control the mind. A controlled mind brings happiness.

—The Buddha

Five years after I started my postdoctoral training at the institute in 1987, I was fortunate to attend a workshop on a new form of therapy, dialectical behavior therapy (DBT), developed by Dr. Marsha Linehan (Linehan et al., 1991; Linehan, 2018) She had added an important ingredient: a focus on mindfulness skills. In addition, she honored that what happened in childhood had a huge impact on what was happening in client's lives, an idea dear to traditionally trained therapists and counselors. I also noticed that she had integrated some of Ellis's ideas, for example, that a client's low frustration tolerance might be contributing to their problems. She called it "low distress tolerance."

Linehan designed a program to help people both accept aspects of themselves, others, and the world and, at the same time, work to change. In the 1980s, she was trying to develop a therapy that would work when CT and CBT were ineffective. She was also practicing meditation at the time. Linehan was worried that suggesting teaching mindfulness as a central part of her therapy would cause her to be thought of as a "complete nut case," but she forged ahead anyway.

The "dialectical" nature of DBT involves helping a client find a balance between being compassionate and accepting of oneself and, at the same time, pushing oneself to learn new skills for managing emotional upsets and interpersonal relationships. DBT focuses on four key skills: mindfulness, distress tolerance, interpersonal effectiveness, and emotional regulation.

At about the same time that Linehan was developing DBT, Ellis developed his concept of unconditional self-acceptance (USA), unconditional other acceptance (UOA), and unconditional life acceptance (ULA). Ellis was reacting to the then very popular self-esteem movement that asserted that praising children (regardless of their behavior) would raise their self-esteem. All children who played soccer, no matter how poorly, received a trophy at the end of the season, something still practiced in some communities today.

Mindfulness, acceptance, compassion, and self-compassion constitute key additions to counseling and psychotherapy. Your working relationship with your client may be the most important ingredient, but learning new skills to manage life is essential, as well.

WHAT CAN YOU DO?

Help Your Client Learn to Mindfully Deal with Metastability

As the Buddha noticed, the human mind is "unstable": "Hard to restrain, unstable is this mind; it flits wherever it lists" (IBIRC, 1993, p. 3). Here the word "unstable" is not used in the sense of being mentally ill. It is used in the sense of non-stable, not fixed and rigid. As we discussed earlier, metastability refers to the fact that things can look stable but not be stable. This has relevance for us as therapists and for our clients. After several days or even weeks and months of progress, suddenly they fall back into feeling very anxious and having panic attacks again, or they become very depressed again or return to some form of addictive or semi-addictive behavior.

The concept of metastability is not commonly referred to in psychology or psychotherapy, but it should be. Change can occur very suddenly and be very disturbing for clients. Their progress seemed so stable, but it was not.

Factors outside us—the seasons, cloudy days, difficult bosses, new job demands, illness in the family, changes in health insurance, pandemics—all have an effect on us. Similarly, factors inside us change, usually without our awareness. Hormones change throughout the day and month and year in all of us. For some, the impact of these changes is much more profound and difficult to deal with than for others.

As I noted in chapter 2, for some clients, I find it helpful to talk about tornados. I tell them that it takes four factors to start a tornado. Many times the weather looks very threatening, but nothing happens. But, at another time, some seemingly small change in one factor may trigger a tornado. During the session the client and I look for the factors that either came together to create a "tornado" or might come together in the coming week to start one. I may also ask them: What factors could you change to prevent another "tornado," for example, another panic attack or OCD episode?

Teach Your Client *How* to Be More Accepting

No matter how you integrate the notion of acceptance into your work with your clients, it will help to acknowledge that accepting self, others, and the world as we find them is a radical idea and very difficult for most people. We are socialized completely in the opposite direction. We are trained to judge and to want things to be different. We are not encouraged to nonjudgmentally observe. Learning and practicing how to observe what is happening around us and inside us without judging takes time and practice. It is as if we are watching ourselves and others and life without any defensiveness or judging or rationalizing, not an easy thing to do.

The RAIN Technique

Michele McDonald, a meditation teacher and the cofounder of Vipassana Hawai'i, created the RAIN technique many years ago (https://www.dharma.org/teacher/michele-mcdonald/). It

Textbox 11.1. Metastability

Sometimes the same stimulus can cause a very different reaction or response.

Imagine dropping one kernel of rice at a time on a table. Nothing significant will happen. A small pile will develop. Then a bigger pile. Then, suddenly, when the next kernel hits the top of the pile, a slide of rice will ripple down the hill, much like an avalanche. Then everything will be stable again, for a while. The stimulus is exactly the same, but the effect is not. What is different? With our clients, we are back to sleuthing. What external and/or internal factors changed that, combined, contributed to the sudden change in their mood or behavior?

is relatively simple to understand and may help your clients with acceptance. In brief, when trouble hits, the following four steps can help:

R = recognize what is happening emotionally, physiologically, and psychologically. What are you thinking? Observe what is happening in a kind, nonjudgmental way. The meditative technique, a body scan, may help here.

A = allow what is happening to happen.

I = investigate what may have contributed or be contributing to what is happening. What may have preceded your client's feelings or behaviors? Notice that this is very similar to the Dalai Lama's "analytic meditation" (see chapter 8).

N = nonidentification. Don't identify or "cling" (the Buddhist term), get "glued" (DBT's term) or "fused" (ACT's term) to any particular thought or feeling. Your clients are not their thoughts. They are not their feelings. They are more than that, a kind of transcendent awareness that can practice RAIN. They can use that awareness to help them do what is in line with their goals and values.

All of us have brains that toss up stuff that is simply not true or a major misinterpretation of what is going on. A client of mine is a professional writer, but every morning his brain tosses up the idea, "You can't do it today." Professor Santos (mentioned in chapter 7) starts off her course with perceptual illusions to help people understand and accept that their brains do not always function perfectly. Then she goes on to more complex situations. We can observe our brain malfunctioning in other areas of our lives, too, and learn to recognize "cognitive distortions" and "brain lies."

Even some psychotic clients can learn to distinguish what are hallucinations and what are not. People who are diagnosed as psychotic see and hear people who are not actually there. One of my clients who is married, has two children and two grandchildren and has managed to stay employed through many ups and downs in the economy, sometimes has CIA agents following him. When I first met him and had listened to him for a while, I suggested that what he had was like a toothache. He looked at me as if I were crazy.

"Well," I said, "it's very aggravating and it makes concentrating on your work much more difficult, but, like a toothache, it doesn't define you. You are a man who is a husband, a father and grandfather, and a longtime employee of a company. Would you like to see it as having malware in your brain?"

He liked that better, and we used that analogy from then on.

What's the point? Clients are not their brains. All mindfulness types of therapy accentuate that fact.

Acceptance and Shoulding

"Shoulding" is when we look at ourselves or others or the world and think, "This shouldn't be!" Dr. Karen Horney is the founder of feminist psychiatry and a strong critic of Freud. (To her, "penis envy" didn't exist; however, women did strongly envy the power and privilege men enjoyed.) Dr. Horney is well known for her writing about "the tyranny of the should" (Horney, 1950). According to her, "the neurotic sets to work to mold himself into a supreme being of his own making. He holds before his soul his image of perfection and unconsciously tells himself: 'Forget about the disgraceful creature you actually are; this is how you should be; and to be this idealized self is all that matters. You should be able to endure . . . everything, to understand everything, to like everybody, to be always productive'—to mention only a few of these inner dictates. Since they are inexorable, I call them 'the tyranny of the should'" (pp. 64–65).

When we are shoulding, we refuse to accept some aspect of ourselves or others or the world. We then create all sorts of emotional and behavioral problems. Sometimes, when the time seems right and in a gentle tone, I say to a client, "But I think you're shoulding."

Many years ago I was working with a client who his wife reported (and he agreed) had serious "anger management issues." It turned out that the client's mother had been very, very critical when he was a child. She had also been hospitalized in a psychiatric ward several times when he was growing up. Clearly, she had had very serious mental health issues. In the session, he was incensed at her. She had not acknowledged his child's first birthday in any way.

When I gently said, "I think you're shoulding," he shot back, "What do you mean?"

"You're telling yourself that she shouldn't have been a very troubled person, and she shouldn't be one now, either. She was hospitalized four times when you were a child, so clearly, she has been very troubled her entire life."

The next session he told me that he had not liked what I had said, but that he knew it was correct. She was a very troubled person. He was very upset by that idea. I helped him see that it still scared him. The world was too dangerous without a reasonably stable and caring mother. But he realized that he needed to work on accepting that reality. And, in fact, he was working on it in our sessions and between them.

We all "should." Terrible things happen, and we have a very hard time accepting them. Many years ago, Columbia University professor and American theologian Reinhold Niebuhr, perhaps struggling himself with that reality, wrote what is now known as the Serenity Prayer. It has been adopted by AA but has great merit far beyond grappling with alcohol misuse.

> God, grant me the serenity to accept the things I cannot change,
> Courage to change the things I can,
> And the wisdom to know the difference.

In an earlier draft, Niebuhr had written the prayer as follows:

> Father, give us courage to change what must be altered,
> Serenity to accept what cannot be helped,
> And the insight to know the one from the other.

In this version, the focus is, first, on trying to change things. Then, if that is not possible, on working to accept them. That sequence may be more appropriate for counseling and psychotherapy and for our clients. Clients may work to change something in themselves or someone else or an aspect of their world. But if they can't, then they have to work to accept that reality. Linehan chose the term "dialectic" to highlight that aspect of DBT that encourages clients to work to both push themselves to change as they are working to accept themselves and others as they are.

There are times when your client should "should." Your client should not accept what is going on. They should leave an abusive relationship or perhaps look for a better job. In fact, it would probably be better if more people around the world were unwilling to accept certain aspects of their social, political, and economic system and worked harder for change. There are also "conditional shoulds." If you want to be a good counselor or therapist, you should continue to read, attend workshops, watch YouTube videos, and so on. But, when people realize that, for some reason, they cannot change something in their life, then it is best to work on acceptance, what DBT-ers refer to as "radical acceptance."

Acceptance or Acknowledgment?

In trying to help clients be more accepting, initially, it may work better to use the word "acknowledge" instead of "accept." To a client who has been abused by a family member, suggesting that they might do better by "accepting" what happened may sound as if you are suggesting that they be okay with what happened. But what happened was clearly not okay. In the beginning, it may help if the client can acknowledge that what happened happened. But even acknowledging it may be very painful process. As a therapist, you can help them also acknowledge that no matter how they felt at the time, what happened to them was a violation and a crime. No matter how they may think that how they behaved made them somehow, in some small ways, responsible for what happened, that is a "brain lie."

Acknowledge does not suggest "forgive." At some future point in time, your client may believe that it would be best for them to forgive the person who abused them. That is a position that many people may never want to entertain, but others, especially some Christians, believe that it is a critical step to recovering. For them, without unconditional forgiveness, they will continue to poison their hearts with hatred. That, in turn, will increase the probability that they will continue to behave in a harmful, dysfunctional manner.

But others may never want to adopt such a philosophy. What does your client think about this? If they are religious, what does their religion suggest about this issue? As my friend Dr. Scott Kellogg (1993) pointed out many years ago, it is not a therapist's role to forgive. That is the role of a religious leader. However, people may decide to forgive themselves and others. Is this what your client would like to work toward?

The Hula-Hoop Technique

Some people find this visual tool a very helpful take on the Serenity Prayer. They can control things inside their hula-hoop. That is, to some extent, they can control how they feel, think, and behave. However, there are lots of things outside their hula-hoop that they cannot control. If they have had an abusive parent, there may be very little they can do about that. It is important to acknowledge that. It is not easy, but, if they want to live a better, more enjoyable life, it is very useful to acknowledge and accept that some things are genuinely outside of their hula-hoop.

Fortune, Fate, Gods, Randomness?

Mark Cuban, well-known billionaire, has reportedly said, "Yes, I worked hard, but the universe also worked with me. To make billions, you have to get lucky. There has to be something that goes really right for you." According to Leonard Mlodinow, the author of *The Drunkard's Walk* (2009, and nothing to do with alcohol), the science of randomness is barely 100 years old. After Copernicus and Galileo demonstrated that we were not at the center of the universe, it took hundreds of years for most people on the planet to accept that fact. Currently, randomness, as an idea, is similarly foreign to most people. That much of what happens in life may be due to randomness alone is too frightening a prospect. There is nothing one can do to affect randomness, other than prepare for it.

Many clients blame themselves for what has happened in their lives. They "shoulda/coulda" done something different and then everything, what happened, who and how they are, and, ultimately, their life, "woulda" been different. For them, it is very difficult to accept that bad fortune may have played a role. That does not make sense. But if it is not luck, to what do they attribute what has happened? God? Gods? Fate? These are not trivial questions. Is everything that has happened really their responsibility?

Historically and to this day, many people have attributed what happens to the gods or fate. More recently, we think in terms of genetics and upbringing to have a leading role. And very recently, we consider attachment and trauma. What does your client think? (What do you think?) Of course, no one has the answer, and no one will perhaps ever have the answer. But it is important for therapists and counselors to discuss what they think in terms of the role of personal responsibility and "fortune" or God's will or randomness.

In the late 1800s, "unfortunate," not "loser," was the term people used when talking about someone who was really "down on their luck." People honored the role of fortune. Currently, people are not as kind toward others and toward themselves.

Hierarchy of Values (HOV) Exercise

I remember running a SMART Recovery meeting once many years ago. Eric, an attendee, had relapsed again, and his wife was demanding that he move out. Someone in the meeting suggested that a hierarchy of values exercise might help and went up to the chalkboard. Another member asked, "What do you value most in life?" A list was written on the chalkboard:

    family
    children
    my house
    my friends
    work
    playing baseball
    going fishing with my children

When he seemed done, the member who had suggested the exercise asked, "Where does the drinking go?" Eric sat still for a moment. "I don't know," he said softly.

He sat for a while. The room was quiet. Finally, he said, "I guess it goes at the top of the list, but it screws up everything else when it does."

"Yes," several other members of the meeting murmured in agreement. That *is/was* the problem. Eric had many good attributes and did clearly value his family and children above everything else, but alcohol upended everything.

Insight into the conflict between Eric's love of drinking and his love of everything else on that list appeared to help him. But everyone in the group also agreed. Insight was necessary but would not be sufficient for change to happen.

Caution: If you do this exercise, you have to be very careful to make sure that your client or group member does not feel ambushed and, in that sense, not empathized with. Insight must be the goal of the exercise and must be done in a compassionate way or not at all. If the goal is to prove to someone that he is not honest with himself about his drinking, then the exercise will backfire and do more harm than good.

It is also interesting to note how significantly people's lists vary. Here are only two from a recent meeting:

financial independence
physical health
family relationships
doing something to get out of myself, like
   service to others, volunteering
sports, golf
learning new things

integrity
my children being safe and happy
my relationship with my husband
my faith
my job
outlets for relaxation

Grudgingly or Willingly

My friend Dr. Hank Robb (2022), in his book *Willingly ACT for Spiritual Development: Acknowledge, Choose, & Teach Others*, points out that the opposite of doing something willingly is to do it grudgingly. If your client does something grudgingly, they may get it done, but they will probably feel resentful and angry. Those negative emotions, especially if your client conducts other parts of their life in a grudging, resentful manner, will lead them to be quite unpleasant people to be around. The ultimate impact of doing things grudgingly day after day is to injure relationships.

Carla, at age 48, with two teenage children, had been left by her husband for a younger woman. She was depressed, thinking that she would be alone for the rest of her life, and anxious that she was not going to manage financially. To her, her future looked bleak, to say the least. How could she accept her situation except grudgingly and angrily?

Accepting when real-world events come crashing down on our clients ultimately depends on what kind of person your client wants to be for the rest of their lives. An angry, bitter person, perhaps drinking too much? Or a person who accepts what fate or fortune, randomness, the gods, or God have given them and try to create an enjoyable life, anyway.

In *The Book of Joy*, the Dalai Lama, Rev. Desmond Tutu, and D. C. Abrams (2016) confront this issue. How can one be joyful in the face of tragedy and pain? Each person must find their own answer. Moreover, that answer almost always involves a combination of strategies to accept, including everything from various and/or combined forms of meditation to baking to encouraging oneself to be curious and open to new experiences in life.

Mind-Wandering and Its Potential Impact

In the past 10 years, a number of studies have been published focused on mind-wandering. Mind-wandering appears to be a kind of default mode for the brain. Welz and her associates (2018) pinged their participants via cell phones and asked them if they were on task or they were mind-wandering. If they were mind-wandering, the researchers asked them a number of follow-up questions. Based on this research, it would appear that when we are not on task—when we do not have our mind on a task—our thoughts tend to become negative and our emotions along with them. This fascinating research may help us understand why some clients in the evening and alone start to feel bad and wind up engaging in some form of behavior that is not in line with their long-term goals and values.

Perhaps educating your client about mind-wandering will help. If they know that mind-wandering seems to happen to almost all humans, they may be less likely to damn themselves for slipping into dysfunctional behavior. If they know that it is liable to happen, they may be more careful to plan the evening and not wind up sitting around doing nothing. Baking a cake may keep their mind focused and prevent a relapse into depression. As Killingsworth and Gilbert put it, "A wandering mind is an unhappy mind" (2010, p. 932). Other research also suggests that more mind-wandering is associated with more anxiety (Figueiredo et al., 2020). Can one intentionally affect one's mind-wandering? Eight weeks of mindfulness-based group therapy found that mind-wandering, cognitive fusion, depression, and trait-anxiety all decreased, and those changes were maintained at follow-up (Takahashi et al, 2020).

Textbox 11.2. Case—Avi: Breaking Hillel's Rule

Avi had been married to Rachel for 10 not-very-happy years. He insisted that he loved his wife, but as he went on to tell me about things that had happened, I started to get the strong suspicion that she was cheating on him. I thought Avi couldn't bring himself to admit it. She hadn't come home some nights, claiming she had slept over at a girlfriend's. Once, as he was coming home very late from work, he even bumped into her walking down the street with another man. She had seemed quite flustered and had introduced him to "John," an old friend who had just come in from the West Coast. But he had never heard her speak of John before.

Two or three times, I asked Avi if he thought she might be cheating on him. He was adamant. No, that wasn't possible. But he was in my office, tired of her constant fits of anger and tired of her disappearing.

"I'm a little confused," I said, using what some call the "Columbo Technique" (see chapter 4). "You don't sound happy. Your wife doesn't seem to be very much of a wife, and she seems always angry with you. Why are you staying in the relationship?"

"I wouldn't want someone to leave me," he said.

That stopped me for a moment. Then I thought of Rabbi Hillel's rule. I knew Avi wasn't a very observant Jew, but I asked, "So you don't want to violate Rabbi Hillel's rule?" Hillel was the ancient Jewish rabbi and lawyer who first expressed the Golden Rule, saying "That which is hateful to you, do not do to your fellow." (Later, Christians turned it around: "Do unto others as you would wish them to do unto you.")

He paused. "Maybe," he said.

"And you believe it's a good rule, correct?" I asked.

"Yes. And I try to live by it."

"So, you can't leave your wife. You wouldn't like her to do it to you, so following the rule, you can't leave her."

We sat for a few minutes in silence.

"That is a problem," he said, with smile. He had a good sense of humor, and I enjoyed working with him.

"Yes, I agree, it's a good rule. And it's good to live by good rules, what I call guiding principles. But we might have to break a rule under some odd circumstance. Is that right?"

"Yes. Maybe."

"I think you should think about it. Maybe this is one of those odd circumstances. I realize you don't want to hurt someone, but this sounds like a painful relationship for you and maybe for her, too. Will you think about it?"

"Yes," he said, sounding sad. "I've always tried to do the right thing by her, but I'm very, very tired of living like this. I wonder what she would do. She's pretty financially dependent on me. How would she live? I really couldn't live with myself if she were destitute and very unhappy."

We decided to discuss that at the next session.

He seemed better when I saw him next. Surprisingly, within that one week, he had decided that he had to end the relationship and that he would support her financially for a year. He had a very good salary, even by New York standards, so I knew money wasn't going to be a problem. But I wondered if she would leave so easily.

"Maybe we should ask her in and talk about how you and she might split up amicably."

"I already asked her. She was emphatic. No. She absolutely has no interest in coming in. But I'm not sure she really understands that I want to break up. I've been so dependent on her for 10 years. I don't think she thinks I would ever do it."

"Have you discussed what you're thinking about with her?" I asked.

"No. I don't think I'm ready for that."

"What do you mean?"

"I don't know. It's going to be very unpleasant. I know she isn't going to want to go. I signed the lease on the apartment. Maybe I should find a new apartment for myself and let her stay there."

"Maybe. What do you think will happen if you say you want to leave?"

"I'm sure she's going to get furious at me and start to yell and call me names and maybe even throw something at me."

"Do you feel in danger?"

"No. I didn't mean it that way. She probably won't throw something at me, but she will absolutely explode."

"How do you think you would feel if that happened?"

"I don't know. I guess I'd be worried that she might never leave. It's just so crazy. How did I get into such a mess?"

"I think it would help if we could name how you would feel. Emotions are usually just one word. How do you think you would feel? Angry, frightened, ashamed, depressed?"

"Probably frightened and a bit depressed, because this is depressing."

"I agree. This isn't what you wanted when you got married. It's a tragedy for both of you. But I think you're talking about what I call 'kitchen depression,' meaning not the kind of depression that you need medication for or need to be hospitalized for. Is that correct?"

"Yes."

"So even though it would be very, very unpleasant, why couldn't you stand it?"

"I don't know."

"But you don't sound likely to talk to her soon. What do you think you're telling yourself to stop you?" I asked.

"What?"

"Well, this kind of therapy hypothesizes that we sometimes stop ourselves from doing things by telling ourselves something like, 'She'll flip out. I really can't stand that. And I can't have her living on the street.'"

"Yes, something like that."

"Well, I don't want to put words in your mouth. What do you think you *are* thinking to yourself that may be stopping you?"

He sat for a while. "I really don't want her to suffer. I think I still love her. She isn't a bad person. I just don't know what to do."

"So, you're very concerned about her and her feelings. You don't want to hurt her?"

"Yes."

"What could you tell yourself that might help?"

"She may also want to move on and find someone better for her."

"Yes. She may. But she still may yell at you."

"She will. I really hate that."

"You know, there are negative emotions that we don't like but are appropriate, given the situation. Feeling frightened and even mad at her for yelling at you aren't pleasant emotions, but can you avoid them?"

"I don't know. I'd like to. Don't you think we could do this amicably?"

"Actually, no. I don't think so. You'll probably have to live with some negative emotions as you go through this. Could you accept that? Have you heard of 'radical acceptance'?"

"No."

"It's the idea that we can't control a lot of things in life. Sometimes it's better to accept what's going on, even if it's very painful. Google it when you get home. See if it's relevant for what you're trying to do."

After two months of hesitation, Avi finally sat down with Rachel and told her that he wanted to leave. As he expected, she was initially very upset and yelled a lot at him. But eventually she calmed down.

I anticipated that there would be more problems at the end of the year, but by then Rachel had found her own apartment and met someone new. It was a much happier ending than I had expected. Avi also found someone else very quickly— another thing I hadn't expected. She was a very lovely person. She was eager to find a good man, and Avi was certainly that. She had a very good job and wanted children. They now have two and seem quite happy.

Insight played an important role in this case. Of course, the fact that we had a good relationship and that he had a good sense of humor helped. Avi's avoiding the discomfort of discussing divorce with Rachel certainly wasn't pathological. No one jumps into such a conversation. That Avi was such an empathetic man made it more difficult. He hated the thought of Rachel being unhappy in some dreadful apartment.

Good fortune may have played a major role in this case, as well.

It was fortunate that Avi had a good enough job to be able to financially support Rachel for a while after they broke up. And it was fortunate that she quickly met someone else. She was also able to find a better-paying job. All of these factors certainly made it less likely that she would try to reestablish the relationship or have to rely on Avi for continued financial help. Finally, it was fortunate that Avi had been willing to be flexible about applying Hillel's rule.

Giving Avi the time and space to work through accepting what he needed to do no doubt also helped. And his learning to accept appropriate but very negative emotions was key.

Chapter 12

Facilitating Acceptance, Compassion, and Change: Emotion-Focused and Imagery-Focused Work

It wasn't long after I started my training when I realized that there were a lot of techniques to help people work on the way they were thinking and behaving but not nearly as many to help them deal with how they felt. This was unfortunate because most people were there because they felt depressed or anxious, and many avoidant behaviors are driven by feelings of antici-pated discomfort, guilt, and shame. Most techniques focus on helping clients think or behave differently in order to help them feel better. Even today, the most popular forms of therapy are CBT, ACT, and DBT, and none of them focus specifically on emotions or mention emo-tions in their names. Greenberg's emotion-focused therapy (EFT) may have been in reaction to cognitive therapy's complete lack of inclusion of an E. As I noted in chapter 2, when Ellis switched over from doing psychoanalysis, he called what he did RT, rational therapy. Then he added emotive, making it RET, because he recognized the key role emotions play in our lives.

"How do you feel about that?" is a very difficult question for most people to answer. Perhaps that is why many CBT-ers do CT or RT more than anything else. However, it is often how we *feel* physically and emotionally that drives what we do. We may come up with an explanation post hoc, but that may only hide the real purpose behind our behavior: to make us feel better. This is true when we stay in bed or avoid doing something by checking emails or texts when, after the fact, we will really want to have done something else.

Many of my psychodynamically trained and psychoanalytic friends look at me as if I am crazy when I suggest that we can change how we feel. Emotions are seen as reactions or responses that well up and over which we have no control at all.

As I noted in chapter 5, at Time 1, I agree. By "Time 1," I mean the first moments of one's reaction to some type of event or adversity, internal or external. Many clients don't know how to respond differently over time, that is, at Time 2 and Time 3. Modern therapists can help clients in at least three ways: They can help clients learn to (1) accept themselves with their initial emotional reactions; (2) identify the emotion they are feeling and then figure out how to respond in light of that emotion; and (3) not crank up or increase their initial emotional disturbance in ways that may lead to behaviors that are not in line with their goals and values, for example, yell at their boss or go get drunk or take too many pills.

Some clients are under-emoting. You need to find ways to help them feel safe feeling intense emotions. Stuffing an emotional response is not the same as observing and acknowledging that that is how one feels. There may even be times when it may be appropriate for your client to increase their anger and to express it. But most clients are over-emoting. That is, they are making themselves even more upset than they were initially at Time 1. Moreover, the intensity of that emotional reaction often leads to behavior that injures their personal relationships and professional lives.

WHAT CAN YOU DO?

Help Clients Identify and Label Their Feelings

Feelings are expressed in English by one word: angry, depressed, anxious. Of course, a client may feel more than one emotion at a time: "I feel, angry . . . hmm, sad. And I guess I also feel resentful."

But usually when I ask, "How did you feel about being criticized by your supervisor?" I get, "I think that it was very unfair. I work very hard." Those are thoughts, not feelings.

It is very difficult for clients to say how they feel. They almost always give us a thought: "I think that it was very unfair." It helps to tell clients that if they start with "I feel that . . ." or "I think that . . ." they are going to give us a thought or a belief, not an emotion. Helping people identify and label how they feel is often a critically important step in learning how to manage emotional storms.

It is also useful to point out that words like "upset," "bad," or "frustrated" don't tell us or them how they really feel. What do they mean by "upset?" What kind of upset? Even "frustrated" is unclear. Some people get angry when they get frustrated and may yell at someone or quit in disgust. Others get depressed and give up. Still others get anxious. Finding out what a client really feels when frustrated can be a challenge.

Occasionally, if you think it will help, write four feeling words on a piece of paper and ask your client to tell you which one is closest to what they're feeling. I joke that many lawyers are cut off at the neck and many computer scientists at the nose. As a result, they can't tell you how they feel down below. But that is only partly a joke. Some therapists find it helpful to have a chart with 10 to 20 feeling words.

Unfortunately, we also have the problem that English and perhaps other languages do not have many words for what I call the "middle." We have words for negative states (e.g., anxious, anger, ashamed, etc.) and for positive states (e.g., happy, joyful, etc.), but we don't have many words for how we feel when we are busy and engaged. How do they feel about their work, assuming it is engaging? Finally, we have words like "bored" and "loved," but they are really words for states of being, and we definitely have feelings about both.

The mindfulness movement has brought the ideas of being grateful and being compassionate and kind into the therapy field. Your client may feel infuriated about the many injustices in the world, and they may be anxious about holding onto their job. Being infuriated and anxious may be completely appropriate, but at the same time that they feel those emotions, they can also be grateful for many of the things that they do have in life. They can be grateful for the positive qualities that they do exhibit. You, yourself, can be grateful because you have developed skills so that you can be helpful to people.

On the other hand, in her wonderful book *Bright-Sided*, Dr. Barbara Ehrenreich (2009) argued that it is crazy to try to put a positive spin on negative events. She had been diagnosed with breast cancer and a friend suggested that it "was the best thing that could have happen to her." She detested such a Panglossian approach. But at the same time, one can be grateful for having the friend, and rereading a list of reasons to be grateful may help a client feel more hopeful and less depressed.

Fromm (1967), in his book *The Art of Loving*, points out that it is better to see love as a verb and not a noun. As a noun, we may endlessly go "looking for love." As a verb, throughout our lives, with different people—partners, children, friends—we can study how to do it well. As Fromm's title indicates, he suggests that love is an art. As an art, it needs to be given time and attention, and it needs to be practiced. The same is true of feeling grateful. It requires time, attention, and practice.

Help Clients Identify Their Emotional Goals

With regard to feeling better, it may be useful to ask a client how they would prefer to feel, instead of depressed, anxious, hopeless, shameful, and so on.

Sometimes when I ask clients what they would like to feel, they say "nothing."

"That's a nice idea," I respond. "But I'm afraid that is not an option. Whether we like it or not, we always feel something."

One time, someone who had moved to New York to work in fintech answered, "Calm, happy, and relaxed." I noted that most people who wanted to feel that way lived outside of cities. In fact, for thousands of years, most monasteries were built outside of cities. I didn't add—because it was too early to do so—that fintech, while exciting, is not for people who seek to spend their day calm and relaxed.

No doubt, sometimes the best approach is to just sit with and accept an emotion. But that may leave a client feeling completely hopeless, helpless, and trapped. Even if, at times, it is very difficult to change how we feel, it can be done. People do not have to be victims of how they feel. But it may take considerable time and work.

Help Clients Accept Appropriate Negative Emotions

If people make a mistake, it is quite common to feel regretful. The mistake is not in line with their goals and values. For the same reasons, if they forget an appointment or arrive late, they may feel irritated and embarrassed. These are also not pleasant emotions. They create discomfort. But they fit the situation. Trying to get rid of them may lead clients to do things, such as procrastinate, watch a video, or smoke a joint, which makes matters worse in the long run.

Teaching your clients to make a distinction between functional (helpful, in line with their goals and values) emotional responses and dysfunctional (unhelpful) emotional responses can be very therapeutic. In fact, beginning to feel panicky (or intense anxiety) instead of just worried and reasonably anxious can be a signal that they have slipped over a line between thinking rationally and flexibly about a situation and thinking in a demanding, rigid manner: *I must do well. It would be awful if I screwed up.*

A thermometer may tell us that we have a fever and that may mean that we have an infection. Annoying as that may be, the thermometer and fever are useful and helpful. They tell us that we should change our behavior. We should get more rest, drink more liquids, and maybe take some medication or go to a doctor. Intense anxiety may not be pleasant, but it may signal a need to take some action, for example, to do a mindfulness exercise or some DDB, deep diaphragmatic breathing.

Sitting With

Mindfulness practitioners recommend a radically different approach from what most clients have been raised to do. Many clients have been taught—and have learned and even overlearned—to ignore their emotions or stuff them down very deeply and get on with it, or try to get rid of them, perhaps by cutting themselves, drinking, or binge-watching TV. At times, it is better to sit and observe an emotion rather than try to make it go away, change it, or numb oneself to it. The RAIN technique suggests (see chapter 11) an alternative: Recognize the emotion. Allow it to exist. Investigate it. Don't identify with it (nonidentification).

Shame Attacks

For my clients, I make a distinction between guilt and shame. Not everyone will agree, but I describe guilt as what you feel when you behave badly. For example, you lose your temper with someone you love, and you feel guilty. Shame is very different. It is a feeling about your totality. You lose your temper and feel like a totally worthless human being. You are beyond hope. Shame cuts you off at the knees. In contrast, guilt may motivate you to figure out how to change your behavior and how to avoid repeating it.

Shame is as "toxic" as John Bradshaw (1988) suggested many years ago. Ellis believed that shame was so toxic that many people did all kinds of things to avoid even the possibility of feeling shame. As a result, he created his Shame Attack exercise. Most often, shame attacks were given as homework assignments. In training, everyone had to do at least one. After giving the assignment, Ellis gave several examples, some very humorous but others simply ideas of doing something that would cause people to feel shameful and help them learn to better handle the associated discomfort; for example, if they are perfectionists, ask them to come late to the next session.

You will find that clients often come up with things that they would consider shameful that you would probably never think of. During an all-day group workshop, one member decided at lunchtime to go to the fancy Fifth Avenue store Hermès and ask someone to show him a number of items and then to leave without buying anything. To him this was very shameful behavior— taking a salesperson's time and then leaving without buying something—and, in fact, he did not succeed. He bought the least expensive item in the store, a scarf for $75.00. When he came back after lunch with the scarf, the group sent him back to return it. He did, and he survived.

Shame attacks are not a new technique. Haleh Liza Gafori (2022), relates how Sham, an older, vagabond-like mystic guide and mentor to Rumi, the great Persian poet and mystic in the 13th century, prodded and pushed him to change his thinking about thinking and about what we would call his self and self-image. According to Gafori, one time Sham told Rumi to carry a bottle of wine—drinking alcohol is forbidden in Islam and Rumi was a leader in his community—in plain sight through the streets to his home. Much more recently, Jason Comely's rejection therapy (https://www.rejectiontherapy.com) is based on the same idea.

Imagery

Most forms of CBT focus on what people might be thinking or saying to themselves. Not as much attention, if any attention at all, is given to the images that may be fueling the anxiety, depression, or addictive behaviors. In contrast, Lazarus made "imagery" one of the seven key elements of his multimodal therapy and some researchers have focused on the role of imagery in psychotherapy (Sheikh, 2020; Skottnik & Linden, 2019). Olympic ice-skating dancers have used imagery to improve their performance, and Buddhists, especially Tibetan Buddhists, have used images for thousands of years. Devotees intentionally focus on specific aspects of an image, or, at times, a mandala, to aide in their spiritual development.

Textbox 12.1. Case—Harry: Inference Chaining

Many thoughts involve images, not words. My client Harry hated to make cold calls. He had had a panic attack after making calls one day at the office, and he had stayed home from work sometimes just to avoid the situation. But he was going to lose his job if he was unwilling to make such calls. I asked him to do an exercise with me called "inference chaining," and he agreed. I also asked him to let the irrational, "wacky" part of his brain have its say and, as much as possible, not to come in with more reasonable thoughts. (Harry had already told me that he preferred "wacky" when he was thinking about thoughts that his brain tossed up that did not make sense and were not helpful. Sometimes I suggest "silly," "nutty," or even "crazy," but I always ask my client which one they prefer.) He agreed, so I asked, "So what do you see happening if you call someone from the cold-call list?"

"They'll blow me off."

"And then what? What's the worst-case scenario? Try to let the wacky part of your brain talk, just this once."

"I'll refuse to make another one. It's too painful to be rejected like that. I might have a panic attack."

"And let's suppose you do. I don't think you would, but you might and, anyway, we're here safe in my office. Then what would happen?"

"I'd just sit at my desk like a dummy, and I'd get fired."

"Well, let's suppose that happens. You sit at your desk like a dummy, you don't make any cold calls, and you get fired. Then what? Worst-case scenario."

"Then, I don't know, I wouldn't have a job and my wife would leave me."

"And?"

"I couldn't afford our house and I'd have to find an apartment and the children would refuse to come stay with me, and I think I'd go insane."

"Well, I don't think so, but just for this exercise, let's go a few steps further. What do you see happening then?"

"I'd get really depressed like I was in college, and I wouldn't be able to leave the apartment. I wouldn't be able to keep the apartment. I guess I'd be homeless and have to live on the street. And my children wouldn't respect me."

"And?"

"Isn't that bad enough!"

He looked like he might start to cry.

"Yes, of course. That is very, very bad. But I don't think that's going to happen."

We sat for a few minutes quietly.

"You know, I don't think you should make any cold calls if that is going to happen," I said with a smile.

"What?!"

"If your brain thinks that's going to happen, I'm not surprised at all that cold calls make you freeze. That is absolutely horrifying. To be abandoned by your wife and not respected by your children."

Again, we sat for a moment.

"God forbid," I said, and smiled. "No cold calls!"

He looked at me and smiled, too. Then he said, "But they wouldn't abandon me. That's wacky."

"I know, but that's what a part of your brain thinks will happen, and it's trying to protect you against that horrifying scenario. Let's look at each of the links in the chain. We can't just leave you there with those terrifying thoughts. If you lost your job—and that's a big if—now you're saying that your wife wouldn't leave you?"

"Yes. She's not like that. She wouldn't leave me."

"And if you lost your job, would you never get another one?"

"I don't know. It's a tough market out there."

"Yes, I know, but you've known other people who have lost their job and they've gotten a new one, correct. You've even lost your job twice, and you got new ones, correct?"

"Yes."

"Okay. So we're going to look at each of the links. Right now it's too scary to make a cold call, at least for you. There is too much to lose . . . your wife, your children's respect, everything!"

"I don't think that would really happen."

"But a part of your committee, your brain, does. Think about it during the week and we'll work on another link or two next week. In fact, think about which links we should focus on."

"But they're so wacky."

"Yup. I agree. But unless we talk about them, they will scare the wits out of you, and you won't make cold calls."

"Okay."

"Okay."

Actually, as sometimes happens, just airing out the "wacky" ideas helped Harry so much that he started to make some cold calls. Things don't always work out so nicely, but sometimes they do.

A scoping review of 320 RCTs by Giacobbi et al. (2017) reported that 77% of the studies found positive results from the use of guided imagery with a wide variety of problems, including anxiety, pain, and sports skills enhancement.

If you can teach and coach guided relaxation, some clients will find it much more helpful than self-talk or other ways that they have tried to calm themselves down. Once clients have learned this technique, they can use it effectively in many settings if they start to get anxious. And once they have practiced it for a while, they can do it quite rapidly, and other people around them will not be aware that they are doing it.

Start by talking quietly and calmly, and say: "Think of a place and time when you were relaxed, the way you would like to be much more often and without any drugs or alcohol." If they can't think of a place and time, and, sadly, some clients have never, ever relaxed—they have been perpetually on alert and tense—then have them invent or imagine a place and time. Assuming they can remember a time when they were relaxed and calm the way they would like to be more often, find out the exact place and time. Ask them to describe what they see and hear. When you guide them, use this information to make the experience more real for them.

The last time I did this was with a client who remembered one time being wonderfully relaxed and calm on a beach on Long Island at sunset.

"Start with your feet. Imagine the way your feet felt that day while you were sitting on the beach on Long Island at sunset. Try to get your feet to feel the way they felt that day when you were relaxed and calm on the beach. Work from the inside out, from your bones to the surface of your skin. Try to remember how your feet felt and reevoke that feeling."

I stayed quiet for a few seconds and then continued: "Now do the same thing with your hands. Focus on your hands and fingers. Get them to feel the way they felt that day, calm and relaxed." I also kept my voice very calm and relaxed, speaking a bit more slowly than I ordinarily speak.

"Now go back to your feet and make sure they are relaxed and calm like on that day, while you sat enjoying the warmth and the air and the sunset."

"Now go back to your hands and help them relax."

"Now work on your legs. Reevoke, from the inside out, how they felt that day."

I paused to let him work on his legs and hands and feet.

"Now move to your arms. Get them to feel the way they felt that day when you were calm and relaxed on the beach."

"Now move to your shoulders."

I continued working this way with him, moving his attention from his shoulders to his buttocks, back to his shoulders, then to his back and neck, his head and forehead and then to his eyes and jaw, and then into his chest and, lastly, his stomach.

It may take 10 minutes. While practicing at home, initially, it may take someone as long as 30 minutes. But subsequently, they can learn to do it in a minute or less.

I continued: "Take your time. Let yourself sit on the beach for a while, calm and relaxed, the way you would like to be more often. Check each part of your body again. Your feet, hands, legs, arms, shoulders, neck, forehead, face, and core."

After a few minutes, I said, "Open your eyes. How able were you to do that, between 0 and 100%?"

Some people will say 85%, some 65%, and some only 30%. This will give you additional information into how tense and hypervigilant they are.

If they seem to have liked the experience, encourage them to practice this exercise at least once per day. If they're having to have an operation, doing this exercise in the pre-op room will help them make the experience less noxious. It can help them feel more in control. Most hospitals continue to be oblivious to the psychological impact of their rules and their environment. They strip people of their clothes and belongings, and then have them sit all alone in a cold room in a flimsy gown. It is as if hospitals want to make people more anxious. This imagery exercise helps people move their attention away from frightening images and thoughts to a calmer, more peaceful spot. In one sense, they are no longer in the inhospitable hospital room. They have also regained a modicum of control, which may help them feel more agentic and less helpless.

There are now lots of guided imagery apps that your client can download, including those offered by CALM and Headspace. As with DDB, your client can directly affect their nervous system in this way.

Physicalizing

Hayes and Smith's (2005) *Get Out of Your Mind & Into Your Life* has many exercises to help people put some distance between an idea or feeling that they are having and their sense of self. Many of them involve imagery. Physicalizing (pp. 137–140) can also help your client investigate a feeling.

Textbox 12.2. Case—Sally: Calm or Upbeat and Alert?

In some situations, your client should *not* try to calm down.

Many years ago, I learned that from a TV coach. Consequently, when a client tells me that they can't calm down before a presentation, I say, "Well, you shouldn't try to calm down. That doesn't make any sense. You should try to be alert, bright, and ready to answer any question you're asked. We need to get you excited, ready to be there. You have something to say! That's why you were asked to make the presentation."

Working with Sally, I asked her, "Can you think of a time when you are happy and really enjoying yourself?"

"Yes, when I'm skiing," she said.

"When are you having fun skiing, you still have to be alert and careful, correct?"

"Yes," he said.

"Can you imagine being pumped, upbeat, smiling, having fun?" I asked.

"Yes."

"What time is it? Where are you?"

"It's two o'clock in the afternoon. By that time, I'm loosened up and usually skiing my best. I'm on an intermediate slope, skiing with my kids, on a trail in a Connecticut ski place."

"Great," I answered. "So, before making the presentation, I want you to go there multiple times and imagine yourself skiing and having fun. But you need to remember that someone in the audience, perhaps your boss, for some reason, may want to make you look bad. You need to be alert like you always are when you are skiing, but still upbeat.

"And what's nice about this imagery," I add, "is that if you fall, it's not the end of the world. It's not what you want, but if it happens while you're skiing, what do you do?"

"I get up, collect myself, dust the snow off, and then I get going again, usually a little shaken, but trying to enjoy the skiing and not fall again," she answered.

"Yes. That's what you want. If you say something or something doesn't go well during the presentation, you're going to get back on track and finish what you intended to say. It's not the end of the world. I assume you don't feel ashamed and mortified when you fall skiing, is that correct?"

"Yes."

"So that's the attitude you need to have when you practice this exercise every day before the show. Upbeat, smiling, ready to go! Imagine yourself falling and getting up—not ashamed or mortified—recovering your nerve and going on. Okay?"

She practiced the presentation every day and when she walked up to the podium, she was smiling and ready, as if she were ready to go down the slope, in the afternoon.

If your client tries to calm down before going on a job interview or talking to a boss about a raise and they can't, a vicious feedback loop may start: "OMG. I'm so tense. I have to calm down." Using a form of self-guided imagery in which they are upbeat and feeling good can work much better for them than trying to calm down.

In the exercise, the client identifies a target feeling, for example, anxiety in their gut or core. They are asked to close their eyes and to put the feeling outside of themselves on the floor or on a street about four or five feet in front of them. Then they are asked to describe the feeling in terms of the following nine physical dimensions:

Shape: "If this target had a shape, what shape would it be?"
Size: "If this target had a size, how big would it be?"
Color: "If this target had a color, what color would it be?"
Power: "If this target had power, how powerful would it be?"
Weight: "If this target had weight, how much would it weigh?"
Speed: "If this target had speed, how fast would it go?"
Surface texture: "If this target had surface texture, what would it feel like?"
Internal texture: "If this target had internal texture, what would feel like inside?"
Water volume: "If this target could hold water, how much volume would it hold?"

Then the client is encouraged to meditate on the object for a moment. Can they accept the object without trying to get rid of it or push it away or avoid it? That is, can they accept it as it is?

If there are aspects of the object that have "sticky negative reactions," they are encouraged to take that reaction and put it out in front of them in a similar manner and to go through the exercise with that feeling.

The final step asks the client to take the feeling back inside of them and to notice how it may have changed, for example, in size, weight, or power.

If a client tries this exercise with a feeling that they try to ignore, push away, avoid, or anesthetize, they may notice that the feeling/"object" has become less toxic, lighter, and less powerful and that they are more able to sit with it within them.

Rational Emotive Imagery (REI)

Emotional responses come on so quickly that they often overwhelm our abilities to respond in a functional manner. REI, originally created by Dr. Maxie Maultsby (1971), gives clients a way to practice, at their discretion and time and place, how to respond better. A key element in REI is to have the client initially reevoke as strongly as possible the emotional responses and behavioral responses to an imagined situation. Then they practice working to change their response to something less intense and dysfunctional, that is, more in line with their goals and values.

When I went for postgraduate training, I was asked to observe the Friday night workshop that Ellis ran every week that he was in New York. Ellis was a 1930s socialist, and along with George Miller, one of the founders of cognitive psychology, strongly believed in giving psychology away. His Friday night demonstrations with two volunteers also gave people a chance to observe Ellis's form of therapy in action, and it often motivated them to start therapy. Ellis was partly an entertainer, frequently cracking jokes and using four-letter words. I was not a fan. However, I realized that some people came every Friday night, partly to watch Ellis and partly to socialize afterward with the other attendees and enjoy the coffee and donuts. All for $5.00!

By the time Ellis suggested REI, he had already worked with the volunteer, so he was aware of the client's issues. In one case, the volunteer reported such intense anxiety that they could not ask their boss for a promotion. Once a reasonable emotional goal was determined, Ellis started by saying, "Okay, close your eyes and see yourself in the situation and get yourself really, really anxious, and when you have, raise your finger."

When the volunteer raised their finger, he said, "Okay. Now change your very anxious feelings to just concern, and when you do that, raise your finger."

More than once I watched as a volunteer struggled to change their panic or rage or hopelessness into something that they could live with and work with. Often they would say, "I can't."

Ellis's response was immediate: "Oh, yes, you can. Yes, you can. Keep working at it."

Eventually, the volunteer hesitantly put up their finger.

Then Ellis said, "Great. How did you do *that*?"

The volunteer said, "I told myself that I wasn't going to die, and I imagined myself speaking to my boss anyway."

"And how did you try to *feel* when you did that?" Ellis asked.

"I tried to feel concerned and worried but not panicky. It *is* important that I ask for a promotion if I want to move up in the company."

"That's correct. If you want to *do* better you had better *push* yourself and practice REI *a lot* so that you can *stand* feeling uncomfortable but not panicky and ask for the g-d-dammed promotion (*big* smile). Very good."

REI helps because clients can practice multiple self-exposures at their own convenience in a safe setting. Having to ask for a promotion does not happen often, but REI lets clients practice on their own as often as they think necessary. No doubt, we are conditioned, and sometimes in annoying ways that may have happened many years ago. REI works because it slowly and eventually replaces the old, undesirable conditioning with new, more functional conditioning. It offers a client a way to recondition themselves (to rewire their brains if they prefer that way of thinking) so as to respond in a more functional manner. Thirty years ago, in professional sports, skaters started to adopt the idea that they could improve by imaging (imagining) themselves doing their entire skating routine again and again. Such imaging is now standard among many professional skaters. Basketball players practice free throws in a similar fashion, sitting in a chair.

Chairwork

Chairwork is an experiential technique, developed by Perls, one of the founders of Gestalt therapy. Greenberg correctly describes chairwork, both two chairwork and empty chairwork, as a psychodramatic technique that is very effective at helping people express and work through their feelings, especially intense, unresolved feelings about significant others in their life. Experiential work relies on experiences to provide insight into a problem and that insight, in turn, theoretically, may help resolve a problem. Chairwork is also based on the idea of the multiplicity of selves. The metaphor "the committee" also suggests to clients that they have many conflicting voices pushing them to do X or Y. Most clients experience internal conflict every day, often on an almost hourly basis, and may be in therapy partly because of such conflict. A mature, goal-focused self may be sufficiently positive and confident to take the necessary next steps forward, but, at almost the same time, their brain (or perhaps their entire nervous system, we don't know yet where such ideas exactly come from) tosses up the idea that they can't do what they are trying to do: *You can't do that today. Try again tomorrow.* And they may watch themselves shift from doing a challenging task to watching a YouTube video or answering an easy email.

Chairwork helps people work through such conflicts. The critical part can be put in one chair and the mature part sits and expresses how they feel about being criticized and thwarted.

Chairwork also permits clients to express feelings, often suppressed for decades, toward significant others in their past, for example, an abusive parent or partner. In some cases, after the client has expressed their hurt or anger at the critic, the therapist may encourage the client to switch chairs, that is, to take the chair of the critic and speak from its position. That often helps a client take a more compassionate, empathetic, and understanding stance toward the critic. For example, it may help a client see that their mother was simply totally overwhelmed and exhausted by her circumstances. She did the best she could. Then by switching chairs again, the client can tell their mother how they feel about that. Switching back and forth may help the client resolve the long-endured, little or never expressed inner conflict.

Of course, there are times, for example, when a father has sexually abused a child, when this switching approach may not be appropriate, although, even in those cases, chairwork may help resolve some or much of the inner turmoil. For those interested in learning more, Kellogg's (2014) book, *Transformational Chairwork: Using Psychotherapeutic Dialogues in Clinical Practice*, is an excellent place to start. Chairwork is a powerful emotive tool and can be integrated relatively easily into the way you work.

Imagery Rescripting (ImR)

Imagery rescripting helps a client rewrite a traumatic incident (Arntz, 2012). A traumatic event is somewhat like a video clip, often replayed involuntarily by a client, causing psychological distress. "Rescripting" involves rewriting the "script" of the event with the aid of a therapist. It is a combined cognitive-emotive-somatic technique with a long history. Pierre Janet initially used it in combination with hypnosis, but both were dropped as Freud's version of therapy took hold.

There is as yet no set protocol for doing ImR. In the rescripted, imagined version, the therapist may enter the scene and confront the abuser and protect the child. Instead of the therapist, a client may choose to use a shaman-like, powerful figure to go with them back into the scene. In some cases, the adult client may go back into the scene alone and take care of their child in the scene.

In one recent, large-scale international study (De Haan et al., 2020) including sites in the Netherlands, Germany, and Australia, ImR and EMDR both resulted in equally significant reductions in post-traumatic stress disorder (PTSD) symptoms. Approximately a third of the participants (34%) were on disability. Treatment consisted of 12 90-minute sessions over a period of six weeks. Extended exposure to the traumatic material was found to be unnecessary in both treatment groups and the dropout rate was very low (7.7%) for both groups. Treatment occurred in three phases. The treatment began with the client recalling a traumatic scenario and sharing their "thoughts, feelings and needs" (p. 611). In the first six sessions, the client was guided to imagine a different scenario in which the therapist entered the scene and protected and cared for the child's needs. In the next five sessions, the client entered the scene and protected and cared for the child. Finally, the "client re-experiences the event from the child's perspective with the adult intervening" (p. 611).

Chapter 13

Facilitating Acceptance, Compassion, and Change: Genetics, Neurochemistry, and Neuroplasticity

Our understanding of genetics, neurochemistry, and neuroplasticity has changed in ways no one could have imagined when James, Janet, Charcot, Jung, and Freud were working in the late 19th and early 20th centuries. But humans have long known how to affect their moods with chemistry.

In the *Odyssey*, after her guests had become saddened to the point of crying, Helen:

> decided she would mix the wine
> with drugs to take all the pain and rage away,
> to bring the forgetfulness of every evil.
> Whoever drinks this mixture from the bowl
> Will shed no tears that day, not even if
> Her mother or her father die, nor even
> If soldiers kill her brother or her darling
> Son with bronze spears before her very eyes. (Wilson, 2018, p. 159)

Opium and alcohol were very common in many early medicines, even for children, and Coca-Cola initially contained small amounts of extracts from the coca leaf. When that became illegal, caffeine was substituted. How many people are using legal and illegal drugs is unknown. But almost everyone uses some form of drink like Coke, Red Bull, coffee, and/or tea. This is because they notice the impact of caffeine on their system. It almost always makes them more alert. And, of course, millions still smoke cigarettes or vape (or chew gum or wear a patch) in order to get nicotine into their bodies. Moreover, the environment within which we live has changed drastically. Products to eat and drink—to make us feel better—are advertised everywhere, including while we're pumping gas for our car. Finally, millions of people also chew gum, enjoy chocolate or candy, and eat some kind of salty chips. Each one alters our neurochemistry and is probably ingested mostly for that reason.

WHAT CAN YOU DO?

Help Clients Accept the Role Genes Play in Their Lives

For generations, people have tried to understand why human lives may veer off in such different directions. Today, the majority of people believe that God, if they believe in one god, or the gods, if they believe in many gods, is/are responsible for what happens in life. It was not until 1859, less than 200 years ago, that Mendel and others, including Darwin, proposed that genes play a significant role. It is an important part of our job to help people understand and accept various genetically driven aspects of their thinking, emotional life, and behavior. For example, there is no doubt that some people are born with a more reactive nervous system compared to others (see the Research Note below).

> **Textbox 13.1. Research Note #5: Is Your Client "Too Sensitive"? And, If So, What Might They Do?**
>
> Many years ago, Jerome Kagan, who was the Daniel and Amy Starch Research Professor of Psychology at Harvard University and director of Harvard's interdisciplinary Mind, Brain, and Behavior Initiative, and his associates studied reactivity in four-month-old babies (Kagan et al., 1994). They worked with 247 babies from Boston, 106 from Dublin, and 80 from Beijing. The babies were presented with sounds, smells (vinegar), visual stimuli (mobiles), and, in one part, a balloon was popped behind their heads. Everything was recorded on videotape. Two of the many variables measured were the extent of and duration of body movements (fretting) and the number of seconds of crying after each trial.
>
> The American babies cried on average of 7 seconds, the Irish babies 2.9 seconds, and the Chinese 1.1 seconds. But some babies did not cry at all! On the other hand, some babies cried for 89 seconds in the American group and 98 seconds in the Irish group. Those babies were dramatically more upset than the others. Of course, they grew up! It seems fair to assume that at least in some, their nervous systems started off and stayed very sensitive to outside stimuli. Then what would happen if they stumbled onto marijuana or beer when they were 10, 11, or 12? They might find either or both to be very comforting. I have even had clients say, "I felt normal for the first time in my life."
>
> That is why I consistently encourage clients to be kind to themselves. They didn't choose their nervous system or what happened as they were growing up. And the reactivity of your client's nervous system could have had a significant impact on their life, especially if they blamed and shamed themselves, thinking *What is wrong with me! Why do I get so upset so easily?* instead of *It is true. I have a very sensitive nervous system, and I do get upset very easily. But I'm trying to learn how to better manage my nervous system, and I'm making real progress. And when I can, I stay away from people who think I'm "too sensitive."*
>
> Subsequent studies also showed that being highly reactive could lead to "serious social anxiety" (Kagan & Snidman, 1999) later in life.

Research suggests that approximately 50% of alcohol misuse ("misuse" is the current term, not "abuse" or "dependence") is inherited and perhaps as high as 80% of bipolar disorders. ADHD also runs in families. However, in a family of five children, which child or children, if any, will inherit the problem? To date, there is no way of knowing. Moreover, the idea that a single gene will be discovered to explain ADHD or some other *DSM-5* disorder has now been discredited.

Many clients who have serious problems such as depression, bipolar disorder, and severe social anxiety have great difficulty accepting that they probably inherited the problem. This is true even when they can readily identify parents, grandparents, uncles, or aunts who have suffered from similar problems. Instead, they tend to blame themselves and their "weak will" or "lack of discipline."

Similarly, clients who have problems with overdrinking—drinking more than they intended to drink—have a very difficult time accepting that they can't do "what everyone else does." If they were 5'5" tall and could not play basketball as well as their 6'7" friend, they could easily accept that fact. But they can't accept that the impact of ethanol on their neurochemical system is very different from that of their friends.

Fortunately, we now know that the way genes manifest themselves is affected by the environment. Even one's height is not set by genetics alone. Many of the poor immigrants from southern Italy who arrived in New York in the first half of the 20th century were quite short, probably the results of poverty and malnutrition while growing up. But their children were not. They were better fed and much taller. Your clients may not be able to change how tall they are or the fact that their hair is turning white, but the way genes express themselves—the way a gene is turned on within a cell—during the day is affected by a variety of factors, such as sleep and exercise (Hor et al., 2019). I never expected to write such sentences. We did not know this 20 years ago. Our clients usually don't either.

To date, not much psychological research has investigated how our distinctly different individual tastes for X and Y but not for A and B affect our lives. For some, the goal of making money is very meaningful, and they enjoy using their lifetime doing so. That goal would be meaningless for other people. For them, their goal might be to compose music or write novels and screenplays.

Why are people's likes and dislikes so different? Why do some people like blueberries and others won't touch them? Why do some people like cocaine and others don't? All of this is probably a reflection of our very different neurochemical systems, which may be affected in very different ways by medications, meditation, and other chemicals that we consume (e.g., caffeine and chocolate), and the activities that we engage in that "lift our spirits." How we choose to ease our discomfort and unease in life also depends on our likes and dislikes, that is, how much we like or dislike alcohol, nicotine, video gaming, hiking, painting, running, cocaine, cooking, and so on.

No doubt, some likes and dislikes are due to our upbringing, but many come in with our genetic dispositions. Anyone who has had more than one child knows how early children show absolutely no interest in one thing and are totally fascinated by something else. For therapists, our client's likes and dislikes may be very relevant for a successful outcome in therapy. Helping people accept their "nature" is as important in therapy as helping them accept what happened to them in terms of "nurture."

When working with someone who is having a very hard time changing one or more behaviors, it is important to help them understand why it may not be easy to do so. Their genetic givens (or God-given or both), their likes and dislikes, and their neurochemistry may make it much more difficult to change than it would be for someone else.

Stop Shaming and Blaming

Your client did not choose to inherit a problem like ADHD or persistent depressive disorder (PDD, "dysthymia" in previous editions of the *DSM*), alcohol misuse, bipolar disorder or schizophrenia, and blaming and shaming don't help. It is difficult enough to live an enjoyable life managing such problems. Sometimes, to add a little humor, I smile and say that if shaming and blaming *did* work, I would coach them on how to do it better. But it doesn't. Period.

Evolutionary psychology is loved and disparaged by scientists with equal fervor, but sometimes I explain to my clients that they may have inherited a very reactive nervous system that has been very helpful over the long, long run. That is why they often experience very intense, uncomfortable anxiety, but, on the other hand, maybe they should be grateful for it. That's why they're alive. That type of nervous system kept their ancestors alive. Without ancestors, they wouldn't be here.

To drive the point home, you can ask them to imagine their ancestral great-great-great- . . . grandparent as he walked home with his buddies from hunting one fall evening. Suddenly, he thought he saw a tiger in the bushes way down on the path in front of them. He urged his friends to take a longer route home. They laughed. They called him the equivalent of a chicken and kept right on going. He took the longer path, and when he got to their camp, all of the other hunters laughed at him some more.

A few weeks later, he again thought he saw something in the bushes. He again was laughed at. He again took the long, more tiring way home. But this time when he got to the camp, everyone was crying. One of his friends had been attacked and eaten by a tiger. The point? This spring he will not be able to create new "little worriers."

Such stories are compelling for several reasons. First, they are stories, and everyone loves stories and remembers them. And they make sense. They help clients accept that some of the characteristics that are very difficult to manage now may have been very advantageous in the distant past. At one point in time, the characteristics that we associate with ADHD (attention deficit and hyperactivity disorder) may not have been deficits or a "disorder" for ancestors who were hunters and warriors. Those characteristics kept them alive. They attended to everything around them. They noticed the slightest snap of a twig. And they rarely sat still. On the other hand, although anxiety and ADHD-like characteristics are great for surviving, as noted earlier, they are not good for thriving in the 21st century.

Textbox 13.2. Research Note # 6: It's All in Your Head. Don't Be Too Sure.

Mice can be raised with totally sterile guts. In fact, that's how we arrive when we're born, with sterile guts. Like an alien planet suddenly colonized with new organisms, our guts get populated with different microbes depending on where we're born, for example, at home or in a hospital.

Researchers (Tengeler et al., 2020) took microbiota from people with ADHD and people without ADHD. If mice with sterile guts had their guts colonized with microbiota from people with ADHD, those mice showed "decreased structural integrity of both white and gray matter regions" (p. 1) and were "more anxious in the open-field test" (p. 1) compared to the mice whose guts were colonized by microbiota from people without ADHD. This suggests that neurodevelopmental disorders like ADHD may be partly due to differences in microbiota, which lead to differences in brain physiology.

Another study (Zheng et al., 2016) found that the microbiome composition of people with major depressive disorder (MDD) was significantly different from people without MDD. Moreover, when mice with sterile guts were colonized with microbiota from MDD people, they exhibited depressive-like behaviors.

Literally trillions of microorganisms live in our gut, most of them belonging to more than 1,000 different species of bacteria. The fact that they appear to play a role—perhaps a significant role—in how we feel, think, and behave underscores the importance of accepting that many factors affect how we experience life beyond how we think or what happened in our childhood. It is another reason that we need to be kind to ourselves when we can't seem to think, feel, or behave as we would like.

Educate Your Clients Re: Neurochemistry

Think anything, do anything, feel anything and your brain changes. Now you have a different brain. That is not true for a chair or your sneakers or practically any other object that you know of. They pretty much stay the same. Both your brain and a chair are physical objects, but your brain is more a whirling mass of neurochemicals being spritzed out and reabsorbed.

Imagine that tonight you decide to drink alcohol. The alcohol will change the neurochemistry of your brain. And with *that* brain, you may make decisions that you would not have made with your before-you-had-a-drink brain. You may decide to drink more or go home with someone you don't know well. If you drink a lot, your brain will be changed a lot, and you may not be able to walk well.

You can also change your brain by just thinking about something. Just thinking about getting together with someone you have had a good time with in the past will cause a dopamine spritz in your brain. Initially, getting together was very pleasurable, and your brain noted that and hasn't forgotten. Consequently, thinking about getting together may cause dopamine to be released changing your brain, and with *that* brain you may text the person, even though you have learned that getting together doesn't usually work well in the long run. Unfortunately, the brain does not always get it right. You are not solely concerned about taking care of yourself in the short run. The long run matters, too.

Is Your Client's Dopamine Spritzer Clogged?

Whenever your clients think of something pleasurable, their nervous system gets a little dopamine. They feel better. Thinking about going on a vacation, eating their favorite ice cream, or spending time with someone they like creates dopamine and immediately lifts their spirits, to put what happens in metaphorical terms.

But some people may not get the same spritz as others. Researchers (Zheng et al., 2016) genetically modified mice so that they were born with brains that did not make dopamine. After birth, they didn't move around very much and even with food readily available, they didn't eat enough and died within four weeks. People who suffer from low-grade depression may suffer from a lack of dopamine.

The mice, when injected with L-dopa daily, ate as usual and survived. Alcohol is the fastest dopamine booster on the market; cocaine is equally fast, but I don't consider it "on the market." Of course, both stop working over time, and depression or anger or anxiety come back, often worse than ever. However, for people suffering for long periods with depression, one can understand why alcohol is so appealing. The drug Wellbutrin, an NDRI (norepinephrine and dopamine reuptake inhibitor), is designed to prevent dopamine from being reabsorbed, making more available than otherwise would be the case, but it does not work for everyone.

Clients may choose to take prescribed medications, but they may also try to learn other ways to cope with and manage PDD. For example, professional work that is "uplifting" may be more important for such people than for others. Caffeine may help, too. Given caffeine, the genetically modified mice did better.

Neuroplasticity, Acceptance, and Change

When I was in college, professors told us that the human brain grew until we were 25 years old and then started a gradual, slow decline. Then when I was in my 30s, in a lecture, a professor told the audience that the human brain only started to decline after around 37. Now no one knows the real answer. In addition, we now know that the brain grows cells every day. In fact, about 1,400 cells per day, especially in the hippocampus, an area central to learning and memory.

> **Textbox 13.3. Research Note #7: Do Parts of Your Brain Grow During All of Your Lifetime? Yes!**
>
> Imagine someone who was highly motivated. They studied and practiced hard for four long years. What happened to their brains? The right back of a very important part of their brain used for navigation doubled in size—doubled! Who were these people? London taxicab drivers (Maguire et al., 2000), before Google Maps, Garmin, and so on.
>
> Some people questioned Dr. Eleanor Maguire's findings, saying that it was the stress of driving in a city like London that caused the change. So she conducted MRIs on the brains of bus drivers (Maguire et al., 2006). Their hippocampi had *not* changed.
>
> Now we know that the hippocampi of other mammals and birds that have to navigate long distances also change. And we know that the hippocampi of persons with Alzheimer's lose brain cells as the disease progresses.
>
> Maguire's taxicab driver studies provide concrete evidence that whatever a person is motivated to do may change their brain, especially if they stick to it. More recently, studies (Farrow at al., 2005; Malhotra & Sahoo, 2017; Mason et al., 2017) show that psychotherapy is linked to changes in the brain, giving hope to clients who may feel that they have seriously injured their brain. Of course, after too many years and too much damage, their brain may never fully recover its functioning, but even that may not be true.
>
> Your hair grows throughout your lifetime. Your nails grow, too. Now we know for sure, some brain cells keep growing, too. Do all brain cells? We don't know that yet.

More relevant for clients may be that there are lots of studies (Doidge, 2007; Farrow at al., 2005; Malhotra & Sahoo, 2017; Mason et al., 2017) now that show that the brain can and does repair itself with time and the right circumstances, for example, after a person stops drinking too much alcohol or using MDMA (ecstasy). Often clients have what is referred to as a "facilitating belief." Such a belief greases the wheels to returning to old coping behaviors: *I have so screwed up my brain. There's no point in working so hard to change.* Both of these beliefs seem very reasonable to people who have engaged in a lot of addictive or compulsive behaviors. But they are untrue. It is also difficult for them to accept that it takes considerable attention, effort, and time to affect a meaningful change in the brain.

The Brain or the Entire Nervous System?

Starting in 1991, we gained much more insight into how the brain works because machines were invented that can take pictures of the functioning brain. However, those pictures only show blood flow. They are not pictures of the flow of neurochemicals such as serotonin and dopamine. So far we have no means of photographing neurochemicals traveling through our nervous system.

What about the heart? Many people feel that the heart is a major node of the nervous system and plays a significant role in how we feel, especially toward other people. That may be true, but we have no way yet to evaluate such a hypothesis, although we do know that there is a link between depression and heart attacks and vice versa (Shao et al., 2020).

Finally, the gut has its own separate nervous system, the enteric nervous system (see Michael Gershon's *The Second Brain* [1999]). Cut your heart off from your brain and it stops. Not so for the enteric nervous system. It will continue to move things along for quite some time. Some of the most amazing recent research focuses on the possible impact of the flora and fauna in our gut on our mood and behavior, as noted above. Other research studies (Bercik et al, 2011; Carpenter, 2012) have shown that when the gut microbiota is altered in mice, timid mice became less timid, suggesting that there is some kind of link between our microbiota and our feelings and behavior. What is going on should be fascinating to learn over the next two or three decades.

It should be noted that medicine, especially Chinese medicine, also focuses on the functioning of the liver, pancreas, lungs, and kidneys, but there is little research so far as to how that functioning affects our psychological well-being, although no doubt it does. Dr. Bessel van der Kolk, author of *The Body Keeps the Score* (2014), argues persuasively that the whole body is affected by trauma and that the whole body must be involved in treatment. That may be why psychodrama, play and art therapy, and even therapy with horses (hippotherapy) are sometimes successful when CBT or CPT have failed.

Who Is Observing? The Brain or a Transcendent Self?

Psychology has been defined as the science of the brain. No doubt, a great deal was learned about the brain during the "Decade of the Brain," but the billions of dollars spent yielded very little clinically useful information. Perhaps many readers are not surprised. If aliens from space came down and started studying the computers in cars in order to understand traffic jams, we would think that rather strange.

The idea that the brain does everything leaves little room for any sense of agency on the part of a client. Clearly, that is not a good route to follow. In this book, I have used the metaphor of a committee for the neural networks that affect what we think, feel, and do. When I'm working with a client, I'm encouraging them to observe what their brain is tossing up. Does it have merit? Is it helpful? What is the best way to respond versus simply react?

But I'm also suggesting that another aspect of themselves is capable of observing and responding differently. What is this part? Is it in the brain or some emergent quality of the entire nervous system? Is it a transcendent self like a soul or that part of the self that goes through multiple lives? I doubt we will ever have answers to these questions. But that doesn't mean that such questions shouldn't be discussed with a client.

Most people, including counselors, therapists, and their clients, have a mixed model. They think we are in control to some extent, but they honor that internal systems and the external environment have a very large impact, as well. How does your client's belief system regarding this issue affect the therapeutic problems that you are working on? How much do they believe they are in control and how much do they blame themselves when they do not behave as they think they should? Do they believe in a part of themselves that can observe and is somehow distinct, the "Big I," or the "higher self," Freud's "ego," DBT's "wise mind," or ACT's "observing self?" If so, what do they call it?

Acceptance, Self-Compassion, and Sleep

How much sleep you need is genetically determined. Some people can get by with 3.5 hours but others need 9 or even 10.5. It is very easy for people in the latter group who need much more sleep than the norm to criticize themselves: They are just lazy. Unless they are suffering from depression, this is almost always not true. They simply need more sleep. Helping them accept this fact and be kinder to themselves can be very therapeutic, especially after a lifetime of criticizing themselves and having other people subtly or not-so-subtly criticizing them. If they don't get enough sleep, they will be less productive and more prone to illness, including cancer. Most people who need more sleep are extremely resistant to accepting that fact and try to get by on less. Some form of wearable or phone app should be able to establish approximately how many hours they need per day. A sleep study in a sleep lab may also help.

Textbox 13.4. Experience Your Neurochemical System in Action: Cut a Lemon!

No matter what you think about, your neurochemistry changes. The changes occur throughout your body, not just in your brain. "Everything is connected" sounds trite, but it's true.

To drive that idea home, ask a client to close their eyes and imagine a nice, fat, yellow lemon. Tell them: "Put it on a cutting board and cut it down the middle from one end to the other. Now cut it again. Pick up one of those wedges and slowly bring it to your mouth and suck on it. Now do it again. Bring it slowly to your mouth and suck on it."

Almost everyone can feel saliva coming into their mouths to meet the juice of a lemon that isn't there. Saliva is a physiological change, but it has been caused by a neurochemical change.

Everything we think about is accompanied by neurochemical and physiological changes throughout our body. Your client's back may tighten up as they talk to their boss, and, eventually, they may have chronic lower back pain. Or their chest may tighten and their breathing change, and they may have a panic attack. Anyone who has wanted to run to the toilet just before a major exam knows what I'm referring to.

Chapter 14

Moving Forward, Sliding Back: Managing Change and Metastability

Many people with chronic illnesses have lapses and relapses. (A lapse is when someone returns to a behavior but only for a short time, for example, eats chocolate ice cream even though they're diabetic but doesn't do so the next day. A relapse is when the behavior and all of the attendant behaviors reappear and continue for days, weeks, or years.) Relapse rates for type I diabetes (30–50%), hypertension (50–70%), and asthma (50–70%) are similar to those for drug addiction (40–60%). Problems like anxiety and depression—major as well as PDD—often are episodic. It is possible sometimes to figure out with a counselor and a therapist what triggered the reoccurrence, but sometimes it is not.

Dr. Alan Marlatt (with Judith Gordon), in their book, *Relapse Prevention* (1985), argued that clients should be expected to relapse. Therefore, they should be taught what to do when they relapse. The authors were strongly attacked by many clinicians in the field. They asserted that suggesting that most people relapse—even though the research was very, very clear that most people relapse—was giving people license to do so. Over the years, however, the approach that Marlatt advocated for has been accepted by clinicians. When I started out, the time between a relapse to severe alcohol misuse and a return to treatment was 2.75 years. Now many people acknowledge what has happened very quickly, often in days, and get back on track.

WHAT CAN YOU DO?

What Factors Came Together to Create the Problem?

A fire is caused by three factors coming together: heat, oxygen, and fuel. If your client has lost their temper with their boss, what factors came together to cause that to happen? Learning to be better at seeing that several well-known factors are coming together can help clients avoid a repeat of the past behavior. No doubt, that will give them a stronger sense of agency and help them feel better about themselves and the way they are living their life.

If you want to put a fire out, eliminate one of the factors. Cool it down (throw water on it), deprive it of oxygen (throw a blanket on it or spray it with foam), or remove the fuel. If a client knows they want to feel less anxious, taking a moment to breathe slowly and deeply (DDB) can have a significant impact on what is happening in and to their nervous system. Anxiety can also be reduced by doing an ABC, doing a self-compassion meditative practice, praying, getting some exercise, and reducing caffeine intake. Gaining insight into what happened in their childhood that contributes to the problem may also help.

Resistant or Stuck?

Psychoanalysts have written a great deal about resistance. But are clients resistant or stuck? They would like to change, but they don't know how to do so. Gaining insight is often not sufficient. They need to learn new ways to manage their psychological difficulties (e.g., better emotional self-regulation and distress tolerance skills).

It should also be remembered that Freud initially announced that he had discovered that hysteria in women was caused by their being sexually abused by a family member. Then he turned that hypothesis on its head. It was caused by his patients fantasizing about such abuse. Why does this matter? First, it shifted the blame to the victim. Second, this is why therapy has to focus on dreams, slips of the tongue, transference, and countertransference. What is being fantasized about is too shameful to be talked about directly. Third, it may explain why some patients were so "resistant."

We now know from the #MeToo movement and the ACE study that sexual abuse is very common. Patients may have resisted the suggestion by their psychoanalyst that what they were talking about was not real because it *was* real. The need for free association and other very indirect ways of working goes out the window once the truth is acknowledged. However, clients may be slow to acknowledge and accept what happened, but they are not necessarily resistant. Instead, they may be stuck using ways to cope that worked in their youth but are not necessary or functional now. Cognitive processing therapy for trauma puts its focus on "stuck points" (see chapter 15).

FDI: Frequency, Duration, and Intensity

Clients may think that they're stuck, not making any progress, but this is not the case. They just want noticeable change fast and that is not happening. It will help to teach them to evaluate behavior change in terms of three dimensions: frequency, duration, and intensity. Are they having panic attacks as frequently as they used to? Do the bouts or episodes of, for example, high anxiety and/or depression endure for as long? Is the intensity the same? Most change occurs like stock markets, ups and downs, sometimes with a serious "flash crash," but the overall trend line is up. Clients may not notice that they are gradually doing better. They focus too much on when things don't go well. Some clients may want to track their daily anxiety, depression, hours of sleep, and so on between sessions (Neff & Nafus, 2016). You may want to use a weekly assessment instrument for the same purpose (see chapter 4).

Explain the Stages of Change

As I have already discussed earlier, the Stages of Change model is very helpful when clients slide back. According to that model and Marlatt and Gordon's research (1985), sliding back is the norm. Most change does not occur in a straight line. It is no doubt annoying and inconvenient and at times very aggravating, but it doesn't make things better when clients shame and blame themselves for what is happening. It is far better for them to try to accept what is happening and to take steps to learn how to do better moving forward.

I frequently use a skiing analogy. Someone who is having a ski lesson wants to get down the hill without falling. If they fall, the best thing to do is to get up and try again. Being embarrassed and blaming themselves will probably make them tense and more likely to fall again. Their focus, with the help of the instructor, is to figure out *how* to do better. The goal remains the same: Ski down the hill and don't fall. Doing better (and, of course, feeling better) requires practice, high distress tolerance, and resilience. The instructor will combine a number of factors to increase the likelihood of success: short skis and some specific techniques. Later, having someone sing while they are skiing may help—not exactly an "evidence-based" technique.

In a similar way, when people who are grappling with depression start feeling low again, the Stages of Change model helps them think about what's happening in a kinder, more accurate, less blame-thyself manner. As a result, they can more readily take steps to get back on track. That is especially true if your client is having to manage a genuine bipolar disorder. We still do not know why the neurochemicals in some people change so significantly from one day to the next, but they do.

Similarly, when someone thinks that they'll never have another panic attack, but it happens, the Stages of Change model helps motivate them to take steps to decrease the probability that they'll have another one. Awfulizing, catastrophizing, and feeling anxious about feeling ashamed and humiliated will only increase the frequency of attacks. Doing better in terms of FDI (frequency, intensity, and duration), and then not doing better is what most people go through as they try to change a behavior, whether it be how they hit a tennis ball, how to better manage their experiential avoidance, or how to better manage depression.

Teach Clients About Metastability

How often have you been working with a client, and everything seems to be going along fine? Then suddenly your client has a relapse to intense anxiety, overdrinking, depression, or some other form of behavior that they had been trying to change. Many of my clients are surprised and dismayed when suddenly their behavior changes. That is *not* what they had expected to happen and are disheartened and often ashamed and angry, all at the same time. All of their work, and now look what happened! Often a partner or family member is angry, making matters even worse. When we help clients understand that such changes are the norm, they become better at accepting what is happening or has happened. It is then more likely that they will treat themselves kindly and focus more on figuring out how better to manage the current and future lapses/relapses.

Use MI with Your Client—and Yourself

As the Buddha taught, life is difficult and almost always involves suffering. Although aggravating and at times painful, change usually comes in fits and starts. Hence, practicing motivational interviewing becomes even more essential. Our objective is to help clients change, but we can be understanding when they don't because that happens so often in life. MI helps us help clients when their motivation has been significantly diminished by a lapse or relapse and they are feeling low and helpless and hopeless. If your client loses hope and feels helpless, what are they thinking?

TYPICAL CLIENT UNHELPFUL BELIEFS

1. I'll never change.
2. Changing should be easier.
3. I shouldn't feel this way.
4. I can't stand how I feel.
5. It's not fair (as it should be).

6. No one really cares.
7. Life isn't worth it.
8. I'm worthless.
9. I deserve better.
10. Why do I keep screwing up?
11. Why am I such a failure at everything?

Help your client identify (and write down) the thoughts that their brain tosses up most frequently and/or that are the most difficult to handle, that is, the most triggering. Doing so will help them become familiar with such thoughts and learn how best to manage them (dispute them, simply let them go, or use some other cognitive defusion technique). Eventually they may even become a bit bemused by the reappearance of such thoughts and think in response, *Oh. There you are again. It's okay. I've heard you many times before. I now know how best to respond.* Helping clients make a list of their most problematic thoughts can be a wonderful way to begin to help them get "unstuck" and to drain the power from some of their most problematic thoughts.

Counselors and therapists also need to observe and learn to manage their own unhelpful thoughts. Without doing so, they will get dismayed, clients will see that, and they, the clinicians, will be less effective. They will also become more vulnerable to burnout (see chapter 20).

Warn Your Client to Be Wary of Questions

You may have noticed in the above list that the last two are questions. Many clients do not realize that they have gotten into the habit of hammering themselves with questions, and the questions are usually unanswerable. This is another way of beating themselves up. In addition, questions can't be disputed or questioned.

Help your client, first, to recognize that this is what they are doing. Second, help them rephrase the question into a statement: *Why do I keep screwing up?* I keep screwing up. *Why am I such a failure at everything?* I fail at everything. Statements like "I fail at everything" are more easily seen as unhelpful and illogical. No one fails at everything. (See DIBS, chapter 16.)

Autobiographies, Eulogies, and Obituaries

Some people benefit from writing their autobiographies, one chapter per decade. They may also benefit from writing the "next chapter," that is, a chapter about the coming decade, revealing what they would like to accomplish. Some clients will benefit from writing their obituaries or how they hope someone will eulogize them at their funeral (see the funeral exercise in chapter 8). However, clients from some cultures will definitely not like this suggestion.

Autobiographies and similar exercises may help clients develop a better sense of how they would like to use their time in life. It may help them make their values and goals clearer. Suggesting books may also help (e.g., Bronson's *What Should I Do with My Life?* [2013] and Frankl's *Man's Search for Meaning* [1985]).

The purpose of these between-session assignments is to help clients gain insight into events in their past, core beliefs from the past and about the present and the future, and deeper feelings and issues that may not have surfaced via other approaches. They may also help you and your client gain insight into what has contributed to and may still be contributing to their current difficulties. However, such techniques may not be necessary with many clients and may be a waste of time and energy.

Teach Protective Behavioral Strategies

Protective behavioral strategies come out of the alcohol misuse researchers' work, but they can be very useful in other areas, too. Not all of the following are behavioral; some, like doing an ABC once a day, are cognitive.

For anxiety:

1. Drink less caffeine. Drink "half-caff": make a cup with half caffeinated and half decaffeinated coffee.
2. Exercise: walking, running, rowing, swimming, biking, karate, tai-chi, Pilates.
3. Meditate, pray.
4. Stop every hour and sit for three minutes and breathe deeply (DDB).
5. Do an ABC(DE) sheet once or twice a day.
6. Watch out for mind-wandering (see chapter 11).
7. Use ACT's concept of value-guided action.
8. Some anxiety is part of growing, learning, and trying new things. Getting out of your comfort zone is critical for human happiness. Suggest to clients that they do something anxiety producing but in line with their goals and values at least once a day.

For anger management:

1. Use Glasser's three questions (see chapter 16).
2. Do an ABC(DE).
3. Work on "radical acceptance."

For drinking:

1. Eat before you drink.
2. Drink two drinks the first hour (not half hour) and then, if you drink more, one per hour after that.
3. Drink less often.
4. Start one hour later in the day this week. Do the same thing next week.
5. Measure your drinks if you make cocktails at home.
6. Count your drinks.
7. Alternate between an alcoholic drink and a nonalcoholic drink. Drink a rum and Coke and then just a Coke. Have a gin and tonic and then just a tonic.
8. Tell a bartender what you want them to do for you.
9. Never drink before 7:00 p.m.
10. Don't drink on both Friday and Saturday night.
11. Change where you drink.
12. Change with whom you drink.

Similar lists can be generated for helping a client take preventive action for other issues. In writing or on their phone, such lists will help them protect themselves against a lapse or relapse.

Motivational Between-Session Work

It is always demotivating to slide back. Everyone needs help reminding themselves why they are doing the hard work that they're doing. One or more of the following may help.

CBA (Cost–Benefit Analysis aka Decisional Balance Exercise): A CBA is a powerful motivational exercise that clients can do at home, with you in your office, or, in a group, together and then one or two on a whiteboard. They can also be done quite easily in a virtual session.

They can be done on a piece of paper folded into four squares or on a computer. In the top-left quadrant, write something like "The good things about using" or "The good things about X," whatever the issue is, for example, procrastinating or binge-watching TV or staying in bed too long. At the top of the right quadrant, write "The not-so-good things about" using or X. Then in the bottom-left quadrant write "The good things about not" using or doing X. Finally, in the lower-righthand quadrant, write "The not-so-good things about not . . . "

Have your client fill in each box or, if you are working online or with an in-person group, have everyone do it for themselves, and then collect some of the results and put them on a whiteboard or Zoom blank document. Your client may say, "There aren't any good things about using," but you can gently remind them that if there weren't any, they wouldn't be doing a CBA. People often forget how much they like doing X, how much it helps them cope, and so forth.

Many people like to do a CBA once a month. It helps them maintain their motivation to change. Once the form is filled in, you can underline the things that are positive or negative in terms of the short term and long term. This helps clients become more aware of the problem: what feels good and is fun to do in the short term sometimes does not work well in the long term.

Finally, a CBA works well because, if the client does it with you in session, they can leave with something tangible in their pocket or purse, something they can reflect on and look at when their resolve starts to weaken.

Positive Attributes: Ask your client to make a list of 10 things that they have done well in their life or 10 things that they like about themselves.

Fill in DIBS worksheet (see chapter 16).

Gratitude List: It is easy to feel depressed and hopeless and sometimes very difficult to feel differently. Your client, like everyone, probably quicky forgets what they can be grateful for, especially when life is throwing them multiple curveballs. Making a list that can be reviewed at such moments can help.

Hierarchy of Values (HOV): Ask your client to make a list of the things that are most important to them. It is surprising how different the lists are that different people produce (see chapter 11).

Chapter 15

If Needed, Dig Deeper: Past-Focused Work, Trauma, and Childhood Issues

Traditional therapy has focused on the past in the belief that insight into what happened in a client's past would help them do better in the future. This book advocates for a combined approach, spending time exploring and processing what happened in their past, as well as time on figuring out how they might help themselves do better in the future (e.g., the coming week), but also including their larger goals, that is, what they would like to try to do with their life.

As I have noted before, there is no compelling research evidence that digging deeper into someone's past will necessarily be helpful. However, sometimes, especially if you suspect trauma of some kind, digging deeper definitely may be critically important. In addition, some clients come to therapy because they want to understand why they are feeling, thinking, and behaving the way they do. If it helps, you can split a session in two, one half on the "why?"—why they might be having the problems they are having—and half on the "how?"—how they might do better going forward. What new skills and between-session work might help?

As I discussed in chapter 3, each session and every exercise offer us an ongoing opportunity to assess what factors may be contributing to a problem. Because of our current culture, most clients tend to blame something within themselves rather than first considering what factors outside them might be contributing to the problem. Perhaps they do, in fact, have a chemical imbalance or something traumatic happened that they don't recall, but factors outside them, like job insecurity, may be contributing to their difficulties, as well. Of course, there are also clients who always look to blame something outside them.

However, many people first look inward. Why am I so depressed? Why am I such a failure? Why don't I have self-confidence? Once you have looked at possible outside factors—systemic racism and/or sexism where they work, they have to work 60 hours a week, quality day care is very expensive, their husband is abusive—then you can turn to internal factors. You and your client may sense that childhood, as traditional psychotherapy has always maintained, is a key contributing factor.

One major value in going back into someone's past may be to help them stop blaming themselves. The fact that an uncle's sexual abuse significantly derailed their life does not mean that it has to continue to derail their life. When they process past events and past relationships, they may start to understand why they are suffering as they are. It may help them acknowledge what has happened and help them stop shaming and blaming themselves. That in itself would constitute a significant therapeutic change. They may also become more motivated to continue to work and to grow.

TRAUMA-INFORMED COUNSELING AND THERAPY

In the Western world, Jean-Marie Charcot, one of the founding fathers of psychiatry in Paris in the 1890s, appears to be the first person to write about trauma in a series of papers between 1878 and 1893, but the concept of trauma took a long time to become what it is today.

The term *shell shock* was based on the idea that the new, monstrously large munitions of WWI created such tremendous explosions that they caused actual physical, microscopic damage. Because it was a "physical wound," soldiers in Britain were given a medal and disability benefits. However, that started to become so costly that the theory was revised. Physical injury was not the problem. Weakness of character was. Medals and disability benefits were no longer given. Here, again, we have a case of placing the cause of the problem in or on the individual. Changes in the outside environment—tremendously loud explosions—were not to blame. The new way of thinking has lingered to this day.

During the Vietnam war, nightly television broadcasts of the war, including the My Lai tragedy, began to shift people's feelings about warfare that are continuing to this day. For every two military deaths, one person comes homes suffering from PTSD that may endure for the rest of their lives. Finally, the impact of trauma entered psychological thinking in 1971, PTSD being included in the *DSM-III*.

In 1998, the ACE (adverse childhood events) report was published (see the Research Note below). It provided the first clear, scientific evidence of a link between adverse childhood events and subsequent serious problems in adult physical and psychological health. Historically, as you know, many, if not most, people who were abused as a child were told, either directly or indirectly, that what they were experiencing was simply not happening. Parents who complained to the Catholic Church were dismissed, their complaints minimized or denied. And Freud asserted that the young women who were reporting abuse by uncles or friends or their fathers were imagining it. Based on one study, almost one in five women (17.2%) has been sexually abused while growing up, that is, under 18 years of age (Bynum et al., 2010).

A therapist who finally validates what happened, and the enormous pain that trauma often caused and still causes, can help a client take a first step to living a life with less pain and fewer

---

Textbox 15.1. Research Note #8: How Does Your Childhood Affect Your Adulthood?

Felitti and his associates (1998) sent a survey to members of the Kaiser Permanente insurance company. Approximately 17,000 answered. Janet, Freud, and many others had always maintained that what happened in childhood was at the root of many psychological problems. This study provided the first hard evidence that they were correct.

If you have never read about the ACE study, please Google it. The survey asks 10 yes/no questions; for example:

1. Did a parent or other adult in the household often or very often . . . swear at you, insult you, put you down, or humiliate you, or act in a way that made you afraid that you might be physically hurt?
2. Did an adult or person at least five years older than you ever . . . touch or fondle you or have you touch their body in a sexual way, or attempt or actually have oral, anal, or vaginal intercourse with you?

3. Did you live with anyone who was a problem drinker or alcoholic, or who used street drugs?
4. Was a household member depressed or mentally ill, or did a household member attempt suicide?
5. Did a household member go to prison?

If the answer is "yes," you are to put a 1 on the right-hand side of the survey. The survey is scored by adding up the 1s.

The researchers and insurance company were stunned by what they found. If someone answered "yes" to four or more questions, they were two times as likely to smoke, seven times as likely to be an "alcoholic" [*sic*], and 12 times as likely to attempt suicide. But that was not all. They were also two times as likely to be diagnosed with cancer, twice as likely to be diagnosed with heart disease, and four times as likely to suffer from emphysema.

So, what happens in childhood affects not only our mental health but also our physical health, which is no surprise to those of us who have always thought that mental and physical health were interconnected. But here is good, solid data.

And the respondents were not poor, marginalized people. All were fully employed, 87% were white, and 50% were women.

If you share this data with a class of students or a client, it is important to remember that someone might conclude that they are doomed. Fortunately, human psyches and bodies are resilient. But it is important to acknowledge what has happened and that it probably has had an impact. Someone with four or more yeses—some of my students had eight and nine—may want to be especially careful about getting enough exercise and sleep and eating as well as possible. Therapy has health benefits, too, of course.

Note: The results of this study were published in 1998, 25 years ago. Most people have still not heard about it. Carefully sharing it with some clients may be very beneficial.

problems. Insight into what others around these clients were thinking when they denied what was happening may be curative. Insight into the patriarchal nature of most societies and the consequences this has had in the form of abuse may often help, as well. But it will probably not be sufficient.

CPTSD

A different form of PTSD has also been proposed, complex post-traumatic stress disorder, although it is not yet included in the *DSM* or *ICD*. The ACE study suggested that ongoing emotional neglect or abuse could have a very negative effect on a person's later psychological and physical health. Dr. Judith Lewis Herman, who first proposed complex PTSD as a separate diagnosis, stated: "Observers who have never experienced prolonged terror, and who have no understanding of coercive methods of control, often presume that they would show greater psychological resistance than the victim in similar circumstances. The survivor's difficulties are all too easily attributed to underlying character problems, even when the trauma is known.

When the trauma is kept secret, as is frequently the case in sexual and domestic violence, the survivor's symptoms and behavior may appear quite baffling, not only to lay people but also to mental health professionals" (p. 388). Herman also notes clinicians may also misinterpret the symptoms of CPTSD as an indication of an underlying character disorder (http://traumadissociation.com/complexptsd).

Unfortunately, to date, as McDonald, Brandt, and Bluhm (2017) point out, there is no best treatment for PTSD or CPTSD, and a client may be best served by offering them a menu of treatment options, something that is now common in cancer and cardiac medicine.

WHAT CAN YOU DO?

The Key: Supportive, Nonjudgmental Listening

Carl Rogers was perhaps the first person to stress the value of nonjudgmental listening. He also asserted that clients could talk about what was troubling them. The source of the problems was not necessarily so buried and defended against that a clinician could only get at it through interpretations of transference and countertransference, dreams, lateness to sessions, and so on. In that way, he and Ellis, Beck, and all of the other CBT practitioners are similar.

But Rogers used a nondirective approach, similar to many existential psychotherapists. He deeply believed in the innate goodness of all people and that giving clients unconditional regard was "necessary and sufficient." Under those conditions, people could self-actualize, for Rogers and many others in our culture, the highest goal of humans.

MI therapists often talk about the MI "spirit." By that they mean a gentle, compassionate, nonjudgmental therapeutic stance. Without that, it will be difficult or impossible to develop a working alliance that helps clients feel safe enough to discuss traumatic events in their past.

Focus on "Stuck Points": Cognitive Processing Therapy (CPT)

Dr. Patricia Resick and her associates (2016) created CPT specifically for the treatment of PTSD. Their book *Cognitive Processing Therapy for PTSD* (2016) contains many useful worksheets. Like CBT, CPT zeros in on the beliefs that clients developed as the result of a traumatic event or events, especially on beliefs that they and their clients identify as "stuck points." Beliefs may be attempts to assimilate what has happened into a client's existing belief system and are often backward looking in an attempt to make sense of what happened (Resick et al., 2016, pp 113–131).

> *If I had done my job better, then the other people would have survived.*
> *Because I did not tell anyone, I am to blame for the abuse.*
> *It wasn't a rape. It was a misunderstanding. I must've done something for him to think it was okay.*

Other beliefs are about a client's entire self or the entire world. These beliefs tend to be forward looking.

> *No one can be trusted.*
> *I always make bad decisions.*
> *I am damaged forever because of the rape.*

The focus of the therapy, using Socratic questioning, ABC exercise sheets, and other hand-outs, is to help clients reframe the above statements toward more realistic statements.

I did my best. I was the youngest and least experienced person there, but I did my best. There was nothing else I could have done.

The abuser was older and much stronger than I was. He threatened to hurt my sister if I told anyone.

There was nothing else I could do. No one protected me.

Many studies have found that CPT decreased PTSD symptoms significantly and often within a relatively short period of three weeks. In 2007, the American Veterans Administration adopted CPT for the treatment of PTSD. CPT was also found to have worked effectively with Bosnian refugees, Congolese women, and Native American women. CPT via telehealth sessions was also effective, especially as the dropout rate was significantly lower when clients could do the sessions from home and did not have to come into an office (Peterson et al., 2022). Finally, a 12- to 18-week mobile app program, Talkspace (Stirman et al., 2021) showed that using texting was also found to significantly reduce PTSD symptoms. However, Dr. Resick notes that for military personnel, "even among those receiving individual CPT, approximately 50% still had PTSD and clinically significant symptoms. In the military population, improving existing treatment such as CPT or developing new treatments is needed" (Resick et al, 2017, p. 28).

Textbox 15.2. Research Note #9: Can Brief Interventions Actually Be Effective for Traumatic Events? Yes. But Some Brief Interventions Can Do Harm.

A structured intervention, the Child and Family Traumatic Stress Intervention (CFTSI), involving both the victim and their caregiver or caregivers was effective in significantly reducing the number of PTSD symptoms in only four to six sessions (Berkowitz et al., 2011; Stover et al., 2022). Those in the program had a 54% decrease in trauma symptoms and were 65% less likely to develop PTSD than those in a "conventional," supportive treatment program of the same length.

One hundred and six children, seven to 18 years old, who had experienced a traumatic event, were randomly assigned to the CFTSI program or to "conventional" supportive therapy. Each session was carefully structured, used assessment instruments. and involved "homework assignments" between sessions. The first session was with the caregiver(s) who filled out three assessment instruments. The second was with the child alone who took the same or similar instruments and then with the caregiver(s). The answers on the instruments were compared and discussed collaboratively among the provider, the child, and the caregiver(s). At the end of the second session, two kinds of between-session homework were selected from "behavioral skill modules." The focus of each module was on typical problems related to PTSD, such as sleep disturbance, intrusive thoughts, anxiety, avoidance, and phobic reactions. The module skills were reviewed and practiced during and between each session. More therapy was available for either or both the child and caregiver(s) if requested.

Each semester, some of my students resisted the notion that such a short, carefully designed program could do so much good. But the research—many different kinds of research—shows that, in some situations, short-term therapeutic interventions can be very helpful. It should be noted, however, that a three- to four-hour debriefing (critical incident stress debriefing, CISD) right after a traumatic incident may not be helpful and may actually cause harm (Lilienfeld, 2007).

Exposure Therapy

Many research studies have shown that exposure therapy is more effective than supportive therapy. However, there are significant problems. Most significantly, 40% of participants quit therapy, perhaps because no distinction is made between PTSD and CPTSD. Clients grappling with CPTSD may benefit from skills building more than from exposure therapy.

Eye Movement Desensitization Retraining (EMDR)

In 1994, I went to a workshop run by Dr. Francine Shapiro. Eye movement desensitization retraining (EMDR) was brand new. Dr. Shapiro explained that one morning she had been very troubled about something and went for a walk on the beach. As she was walking, she began to look at the ocean and then the dunes, the ocean and then the dunes, several times. Suddenly, she broke down sobbing. Moving her eyes back and forth had somehow released what she was, until then, unable to process. As a result, she developed EMDR. She would ask her clients to follow her finger as she moved it back and forth in front of their eyes. That often helped a client process traumatic memories that the client had not been able to talk about before.

Subsequently, there was an extensive brouhaha among researchers who noted that there was no research to back up the effectiveness of the technique or how it worked. Shapiro produced a number of studies showing that EMDR was effective, but some researchers and practitioners continued to criticize EMDR on the grounds that no one could explain how it worked. Others, however, noted that we don't know how aspirin or electroconvulsive therapy works either.

Subsequently, the importance of treating trauma has become more important, and EMDR has gained in popularity, as has a new variant, Flash. According to its proponents, one of the advantages of Flash is that the client does not have to talk about the traumatic event at all.

A Psychodynamic Basic: Free Association

The original theory put forth by Janet, Freud, Adler, and others was that unconscious thoughts were repressed. Originally, to bring them to the surface, Freud and others used hypnosis and even pressure on the skull to try to push the ideas out, to "make the unconscious conscious." Finally, Freud settled on free association, and the talking cure was born.

As noted earlier, for free association to work, it was thought to be important for the analysand to lie on a couch and not be able to see the psychoanalyst. The analysand could project their thoughts onto a kind of blank screen. The psychoanalyst would then interpret the transferences, countertransference, slips of the tongues, and so on. The analysand could not be expected to actually say what was buried in their subconscious. Those thoughts were too defended against. But hints as to what was buried might leak out while the analysand was free associating, saying whatever seemingly random thought came into their mind.

When other approaches have not worked, you, too, may want to ask your client to say whatever comes to their mind. Free association may bring to the surface material that will remain buried if a standard therapeutic approach is maintained throughout the session. EMDR may work this way. The eye movement or tapping may help people talk about things that they were unable to talk about without some kind of assistance. Imagery rescripting can help, as well.

Adler's Three First Memories

If you do not seem to be making much progress or you sense, even in the first session, that there is something significant that your client is not telling you, you may want to ask Dr. Albert Adler's questions about your client's first three memories (Adler, 2002). Adler was a member of Freud's first group, but he didn't believe that the main drive in humans was sexual and broke with Freud. He thought people were primarily driven to master key tasks in life, from stacking blocks to baking a good cake to running a company.

For Adler, a client's first three memories gave him insight into the themes in a person's life and thinking. Given that a client could remember any one of thousands of different events, the fact that they remember some very specific ones was significant.

Textbox 15.3. Case—Sofie's First Three Memories

A client, Sofie, was in therapy because, according to her fiancé, she always worried. She never relaxed. When I asked for a concrete example, she told me:

"We were on vacation in Florida. We were in the pool. There was absolutely no reason for me to worry or be tense, but he noticed that I seemed lost in my thoughts and, he said, my face was tense, and he was probably right. I very rarely relax without the help of pot," she said, and laughed.

So I asked, "What is your first memory?"

She sat for a while thinking and then she said, "It was a very sunny day in California, and we were visiting some friends of my parents. I was having so much fun. It was glorious. It was hot and sunny, and they had a pool, and I was running around the pool, and then I slipped and fell in. I was only about three, I think. I remember clearly being on the bottom and looking up. I was scared out of my mind! Fortunately, my mother's friend saw me and jumped in and lifted me up. I started to cry and grabbed her neck. That's all I can remember."

I sat there a bit stunned. I knew I shouldn't smile or laugh, but there was something comical about it, at least to me. She had started the session talking about being tense in a pool and now she had just told me this story. It had not been funny to her. Finally, I said, "That sounds really, really scary. It's a lucky thing that you didn't drown."

"Yes. I know. It was lucky. And I didn't bang my head on the edge of the pool either. I just seem to have slipped and went flying into the pool."

"Do you see a connection between that and your tension in the pool in Florida?" I asked.

She looked surprised, and then started to smile. "Do you *really* think there is a connection?" she asked.

"Yes, possibly. Your brain remembers. It's like burning your hand on a stove. Most children don't do that twice. What belief or rule do you think you might have taken away from that pool incident?"

"Watch out. When things are very good, that's when God really whacks you!" and she laughed again.

"So don't ever relax, especially if things are going well?"

"Yeah, I guess so."

"What's your second memory?" I asked.

"When I went on a walk in the woods with my family, I lost my favorite teddy bear."

"What else?"

"My dad and mom got in a terrible argument when I was about four, and I ran upstairs to the bathroom and started to cry. When I came down, my dad was gone, and he never came back," she said.

I sat quietly for a moment.

"That must have been very tough."

We talked about the three events some more.

"It seems to me that when things seem good, you could slip and fall into a pool and almost drown or you could lose your favorite stuffed animal. You have plenty of reasons to remain alert, be hypervigilant, and never let your guard down."

We wondered together, does she remember these three events over so many other events in order to be sure that she doesn't forget, let her guard down, and get hurt again?

It took her a year to gradually process and integrate her insight into those traumatic events and their contribution to her anxiety. And it took other techniques, as well. Insight was critically important, but meditation, especially self-compassion-focused meditation, helped her be more accepting of life and less hypervigilant. Being more aware of her breathing throughout the day, and stopping to take a few deep breaths, also helped.

Repressed Memories?

At one point in time, many people doubted the idea that someone could repress the memory of something terrible that had happened in their youth and then have that memory suddenly come to the surface many, many years after. After the scandals in the Catholic Church, that is no longer the case. However, humans are so suggestible and memory is so creative and reconstructive that not all seemingly repressed memories may actually be true. The damage to the accused person and the family structure may be irreparable. Humans are highly motivated to find answers, and often simplistic answers are very appealing to them. Consequently, therapists and counselors should be very careful never to suggest something that might lead to serious consequences for someone's most important relationships. Let the client guide the conversation.

Establishing an accepting, nonjudgmental atmosphere in your office and using free association, Glasser's three questions (see next chapter), and EMDR, if you like it, will be sufficient to bring most memories to the surface. And the reality is that most people can quite readily access memories of traumatic events.

Dream Analysis

Because CBT is not associated with dream analysis, most clients will never mention their dreams unless they are grappling with nightmares. This is unfortunate; dreams can give us insight into deeper issues that may not have surfaced in therapy. Being a client-centered therapist, I occasionally ask about dreams and if a client wants to share a dream, I think it very important to listen, especially because the analysis of a dream may help a client better understand a conflict that they are grappling with.

There is no room in this book for an in-depth discussion of the various ways that have been proposed to interpret dreams, but Gestalt psychologist Fritz Perls asserted that everything in a dream represents a part of the individual. According to Perls, if a client has a dream in which his mother-in-law is driving a pink Cadillac with a large lady's handbag on the seat beside her, each is a stand-in for some aspect of the client's life and thinking. To get at the hidden meaning of the dream, Perls asked the client to take on the role of each significant object or person. He instructed them to say sentences starting with I, as if they were the mother-in-law, Cadillac, or purse. For example, from the position of the Cadillac, "I'm powerful and everyone wants me," and as the purse, "I'm just a purse. I can't do anything. I just sit here. People use me." For more regarding Perls's method, see *Gestalt Therapy Verbatim* (Perls, 1969).

Posttraumatic Growth

Research suggests (Ogle et al., 2013) that most people suffer one or more traumatic events in their life. Fortunately, the majority do not suffer any long-term consequences, and there is also even research evidence for what has been labeled "posttraumatic growth" (PTG; Henson et al., 2021). The Dalai Lama frequently urges people to think about how one might grow from a traumatic event. However, it may be easier for people to think about how they might grow from a natural disaster like a tsunami than from an attack by another human being or beings. Rape or sexual abuse by a relative or family member or bombings by an invading army may be much more difficult to process and understand and grow from.

Clearly, suggesting that a client might find a way to grow from a traumatic experience would test the skill of almost any counselor or therapist. It would be very easy for a client to feel unheard and that the horror of their experiences was not being acknowledged or validated.

Textbox 15.4. Case—Charlie: Conflicting Committee Members

Charlie had many characteristics that other people genuinely liked. However, he, himself, could not feel good about himself. He was constantly worried that he didn't do a good enough job and that he would be fired. Initially, although he agreed to make a list of 10 things that he did well, he did not do it. He acknowledged that it would probably be good for him to focus more on the positive and less on the negative and that a list explicitly articulating some of the things he did and had done well would probably help, but he came to three sessions in a row without having taken five minutes to make up the list. So we made it up for him in the office.

"I can practically see and hear some members of your committee upstairs screaming, 'You don't understand. There is more important stuff to do. Focusing on the positive is a waste of time. It has no value,'" I said to him, as I was watching his face as he started to write his list.

"Yes. I don't see how this makes sense. Well, actually, I do see, but I am reluctant to do it."

"I think you are scared that by spending time writing the list, we are taking our eye off of possible incoming missiles."

"Yup. It always important to pay attention to what might happen, what might go wrong."

"Well," I added, "That will certainly keep you tense and worried all the time. That's what your wife says you are."

"Yup."

"But she is very tired of living with someone like that, even though she loves you. I think you're very tired of living like that all the time, too."

"Yup. That's for sure."

"So let's talk about what you have done or are doing well, and I'll write the list. Would that help?" I asked.

"Yes. Maybe."

So I wrote the list.

"You are like half of the committee, dyed-in-the-wool conservatives always screaming, 'The world is a dangerous place. We need to spend more money on the military and less on entitlement programs, like Medicaid and Social Security.' You are not going to convince them to give up their beliefs easily. Do you agree with that?"

"Yes, actually, I do."

"Personally, or have you slipped into the real political world?"

"Politically and economically. But I get your point. How am I going to shift the 'balance of power' in my committee?"

"Good question. I'd like to suggest a combination of three strategies. What do you think?"

"Sounds good."

"Well, I think we can agree that if you hold onto to those beliefs and the habit of always anticipating that bad things are about to happen, you're going to go on being anxious and somewhat depressed all of the time. So, a certain amount of arguing back may help. And your wife says that there is no way that your boss will fire you. Your boss has said in many different ways—including a recent big raise—that you are very valued. So, while it is good to watch for problems, sometimes you can relax and let someone else do the watching.

"Second, you could adopt a strategy from the mindfulness folks of observing some thoughts and just letting them go. They have no place in what you are doing at the moment. Your brain is tossing them up, but you don't need to attend to them. You can let them drift away like leaves drifting away down a river.

"Finally, we can also review what we have already learned about your childhood, which probably convinced you that such a constant, hypervigilant mode was necessary for survival. I think it was, at the time. Your seeing that it was *then* but is not needed *now* may give you more motivation to catch yourself and change. I'm not sure insight by itself will do the trick, but it may help you reorganize the committee upstairs. As a businessman, you know, as times change, you sometimes have to reorganize the personnel in your business."

"That's for sure," he said. "Maybe that will help. I still have a hard time thinking that what happened back then can still be affecting me now. Time to grow up! My childhood wasn't that bad."

"Okay, let's assume it wasn't. But you may have adopted some rules back there that do not work so well now: Always, always work hard. Never let up. Danger is around every corner."

"Maybe."

Gradually, Charlie found himself enjoying life more, and even his children said he looked more relaxed and happier.

Chapter 16

Subsequent Between-Session Exercises

Between-session work provides clients with the opportunity to practice and assess new ways of behaving, thinking, and feeling. It is also our best ongoing assessment tool (see chapter 8).

WHAT CAN YOU DO?

Don't Forget to Check

It is easy to forget to ask about between-session work, especially if you start with open-ended questions. No doubt, forgetting signals to the client that you don't really care much about such work. Like many traditional therapists, you think that therapy is mostly about what happens in session.

Dr. Resick, the creator of CPT (see the previous chapter), writes: "Based on social convention or other models of therapy, the therapist may be inclined to begin sessions with open-ended questions such as 'How was your week?' or 'How are you doing?' Asking such questions allows the client to avoid working on the traumatic material, and much of the session could be lost to irrelevant storytelling. Consistently beginning sessions with an inquiry about practice assignments reinforces the importance of these assignments in the client's recovery and helps shape the client toward the goal-focused and active nature of the treatment" (2016, p. 103).

Cognitive Distortions

Some clients will find working with a list of "cognitive distortions" more to their liking than doing an ABC. The following handout of cognitive distortions gives clients 10 types of thinking to look out for when they are cranking up a situation from a molehill into a mountain.

Ten Typical Cognitive Distortions

1. Demandingness—Look for "shoulds" that sound legitimate, but that mask unrealistic demandingness, an insistence that someone, the world or you, yourself, should be different from the way they (or you) actually are. Substitute *preferential* statements and thoughts.
2. Negative exaggeration—Sometimes called "awfulizing" or "catastrophizing." Ask yourself: Is it really that bad?

3. Low frustration, distress, or discomfort tolerance—Some people have much more difficulty than others putting up with something. They frequently think that something is either too difficult or that they can't stand it, leading to "I-can't-stand-itis."

4. Self-downing—That is, self-criticism and self-denigration. It's easy to follow up demandingness, awfulizing, and I-can't-stand-itis with self-downing and self-pity: *It's awful that I screwed up again. I can't stand facing my partner. I'm such a screw up. I never do what I plan to do.*

5. Overgeneralizing—Statements such as *I never do what I plan to do* are overgeneralizations because they aren't true across all situations and time. Try to be more specific in terms of behavior, place, and time.

6. Labeling—A very damaging form of overgeneralization. *"I'm a failure." "He's an asshole."* Such statements usually lead to more undesirable behaviors, thinking, and feeling.

7. Personalizing—Taking things personally that really have little or nothing to do with you. When your child does badly in school, it is not necessarily your fault. When a boss is sarcastic to you, taking it personally usually won't help you respond effectively.

8. Emotional reasoning—The belief that if you *feel* something, it is valid. But feeling something doesn't necessarily make it true. Where is the evidence that because you *feel* anxious, something bad is going to happen?

9. All-or-nothing thinking—The tendency to think of things as all good or all bad. This is a form of overgeneralizing. *Jackie was late to school again. All my efforts have failed.*

10. Discounting the positive—*"I cleaned up the kitchen tonight, but I should have done it a long time ago." "I haven't gambled in a long time, but that's because I haven't had any money."*

DIBS: Disputing Irrational Beliefs

Some clients prefer an exercise called DIBS: disputing irrational beliefs. If someone likes DIBS, I encourage them to do it on a computer. Then, when they feel really awful and can't think straight, they can look at what they wrote when they were more able to handle a situation in the past:

"I'm useless."

Who says that? Does everyone think you're useless? How does thinking like that help?

"People never change. I'll never change."

Where is the evidence for that? Have you never changed anything? How does thinking like that help?

"Life sucks."

Would everyone in your shoes think that? What has helped in the past? What could you think instead? What could you do that would help?

"Screw it!"

Who's "it"? Who gets screwed when you think this way? Has punishing yourself helped in the past?

Why do some clients like one "tool" or technique more than another? As I noted before, we do not yet have a science as to why people like jazz better than rock or blueberry pie over lemon meringue pie. They just do. Perhaps when they first used DIBS, it helped them, and their brain remembers. Then when they go back and use it again, it helps again, so it becomes one of their favorite tools.

Glasser's Three Questions

Many years ago, Dr. William Glasser, the founder of reality therapy (Glasser, 1965), encouraged clients to ask themselves three questions. They may be very helpful when clients are stuck or confused or ambivalent and between sessions. They are so simple. Just three four-word questions:

1. What do I want?
2. What am I doing?
3. How do I like it?

The first question is the tricky one. Very often, people want two things at once, but they don't initially realize that. They want to study for an exam *and* go out and party. They want to win an argument with their partner or spouse *and* have a pleasant Saturday together. The first time they do the exercise, asking themselves the questions, they may hear themselves answer:

What do I want? *To have a nice day with my wife.*
What am I doing? *I'm arguing with my wife.*
How do I like it? *I don't.*

Then, if they stop to think about the situation some more, they may hear: *"She has to admit that she was wrong. I want her to admit that."* If they also pay attention to their feelings, they may become aware that they also want *revenge*, which, depending upon their values, may or may not disturb them.

Then a client has to decide. Which do they want more? Revenge? A nice Saturday? A submissive wife? What?

As their counselor, you may help them observe that they don't like what they're getting. If they want to have a nice Saturday, clearly they have to stop doing what they're doing—arguing and desiring revenge. There is no way out of that. They can't have both.

Learning to use these three simple questions as a tool may help some clients get a handle on some of the craziness in their lives. The questions can help them be more mindful about their ultimate goals and values. Encourage them to write down the questions and answers and bring them in to therapy. Then you and they can talk about them. It is, in fact, often very difficult to resolve such conflicts.

Sometimes it may be critically important *not* to avoid arguing with someone. It may be very important to give up the goal of a pleasant day and try to resolve an issue. On the other hand, conflicts in long-term relationships are not going away. They will be there tomorrow. So your client may decide to enjoy the Saturday and discuss the issue at a later date.

You can also use the three questions to help a client resolve a conflict coming up in the future. Perhaps your client is occasionally getting together (hooking up) with someone and then regretting it later. You can work with them to answer the following:

1. What do I want?
2. What am I about to do?
3. How will I like it (what I'll get) in the long run?

At the time, if they have changed their brain with a chemical (alcohol, pot, etc.), they may not be able or interested in answering these questions. Answering them in advance in session may increase the odds that they will not do what they say they don't want to do *in the long run*.

These three questions can help a client take much more responsibility for their emotional life. The questions also help clients observe and identify conflicts in their lives, providing a tool to help them resolve some of them.

The Three-Column Technique

You may want to start this exercise in session. It also works very well in groups. The directions are as follows:

Take a piece of 8.5" x 11" paper and fold it like a business letter.

Turn it sideways. Label the top of the left- hand "column" Self-Maintenance/Chores. Label the middle column Self-Development. Label the right-hand column Fun. Fill in activities like "doing the laundry," "paying bills," and so on in the first column. In the second column, you might put "going to therapy," "getting my MHC degree," "baking." The third column is for things for which you have no responsibility, such as watching a football game or skiing or going fishing. I enjoy doing therapy, but I don't call it "fun" because I'm ethically bound to pay attention, be mindful, listen carefully, and think.

Participants in workshops and students in my Mental Health Counseling classes usually have three columns filled out in a fairly balanced manner. Sadly, that is not the case for some clients. For example, Carlos's is shown in Table 16.1.

As you can see, for Carlos, life was just one job after another. As he admitted, other than using cocaine and having sex, he had nothing else in his life. Giving up cocaine and sex left him with a boring, unfulfilling life.

in Table 16.2, I have reproduced a three-column exercise done by Sabrina after a year of working to abstain from smoking pot and binge-watching TV and trying to find different ways to enjoy her life.

It was evident to Sabrina, who had done this exercise earlier in therapy, that she now had a more balanced life. You may also notice that cooking appears in all three columns. She has to cook to eat, but she is also intentionally learning how to cook better, and it is fun. If she burns something, it really doesn't matter that much. She might even learn something.

Table 16.1.

Self-Maintenance/Chores	Self-Development	Fun
Work/job		Using [cocaine]
Laundry		Having sex
Pay taxes		
Wash dishes		
Pay bills		

Table 16.2.

Self-Maintenance/Chores	Self-Development	Fun
Making meals	Studying	Cooking
Cleaning up the apt.	Church	Movies
Paying bills	Cooking	TV
Visiting my father		Hanging out with friends
Cooking		

You and your client may be amused—although it is actually sad—that a homework assignment that essentially says "go have fun" is so difficult. Some clients have forgotten how.

I asked Carlos, "What could you do this weekend—besides coke and sex—that would be fun?"

"Well," he said. "I have never finished taping and sanding the ceiling in my kitchen."

I looked at him, dumbfounded. "What?!" I said. "That is the worst job in the world. I know. I've done it. You get dust in your eyes, dust in your nose, dust in your hair, and you have to work over your head. How is that fun?"

Carlos looked at me. He really didn't know what to say. Finally, he said, "But it would be nice to get it done."

"Sure, it would probably make you feel good to see it done. I agree. But it's still a chore and a very nasty one. What could you do to have fun?"

Carlos was disconnected with things that he had enjoyed in the past. He had little reason to get out of bed. Nothing much rang his bell anymore. It's also possible, especially when working with people who have experienced trauma, that they are too afraid to do something "fun." They must stay on guard, and they must do something useful.

Fortunately, when Carlos was a child, he loved handball and stickball. Somewhat reluctantly, he said he would go down to the handball court in his neighborhood and see what he could do. I encouraged him to reconnect with the feelings of curiosity and challenge that motivated him as a child. Could he get better at playing the game? That had motivated him before, and I assured him that if he gave it a chance, it would motivate him again.

Note: A simpler version of this exercise is used by British SMART Recovery groups. Participants are urged to do at least one purposeful thing, one practical thing, and one pleasurable thing each day.

Value Clarification Exercises

In chapter 3, we noted the critical importance of hope. Hope is always future oriented. Without hope, people remain stuck. Many of my clients are initially quite hopeless. However, they are in my office or group, so there must be a glimmer of hope somewhere. Clarifying their values and desire to achieve goals, which they may have had since childhood, is often very therapeutic. For example, in a group or in an individual session, asking people to write an answer to the following question may help: If you hit the $35 million lottery, what would you do?

The key is to explore what they dream of doing after they have resolved all of the short-term financial needs of their family and friends (i.e., they have paid off all of the mortgages and student loans of everyone they care about). Then what? What would they do?

In each case, you are trying to help them remember or uncover what they really would like to do. A few clients may come up with totally unrealistic ideas, but even this is illuminating for you, the therapist. Many, however, will list quite doable things. I remember one time working with a young construction worker who had gotten thrown in jail several times because he started fights in bars. His uncle sent him for therapy, which was unusual for that time, but it happened. He was a pretty upset, disgruntled young man, but he was making $26.00 an hour driving a backhoe, which was great money at that time, and he was good at it. He had grown up in a pretty crazy household, had not gone to a good high school, and the other kids in the neighborhood did not have very high aspirations. Fortunately, he wanted to do more. He was not happy working hard all day, then going to a bar at 4:00 in the afternoon, and then getting drunk, in fights, and thrown in jail. When I asked him the "35-million-dollar question," he thought for a while and then said, "I'd go on vacation to Colorado, I'd buy a house, and I'd take flying lessons. I'd like to become a pilot."

Clearly, with his wages, as long as he didn't drink so much and give the rest to lawyers, he could do all three.

"You could do all three, you know," I said.

He looked doubtful . . . and that's when real therapy began.

CheckUp & Choices

If you ask, you may find out that your client is concerned about not only their overeating and overspending but also about their overdrinking. Overdrinking, like overeating, means that you drink more than you intend to drink, and that may be something your client would like to stop. CheckUp & Choices (https://checkupandchoices.com) offers clients a way to anonymously assess the seriousness of their alcohol or drug use. They may also sign up for a program that research has shown helps people cut down and/or stop completely, if that is what they decide they want to do.

Wanting Another Now

Linehan introduced the idea of "radical acceptance" into psychotherapy, that is, practicing accepting exactly what is. A while back, someone introduced me to the concept of "wanting another now." They said, "You want another now," and I asked, "What do you mean by that?"

"You want another now. It's a Buddhist expression. You won't accept what is right now. You could try not wanting another now and see what happens."

I have had similar conversations with some of my clients. In some situations, and with some clients who are ready, what will be most helpful is accepting what is, period. Some clients are motivated enough—perhaps because they have gone through so much—that they are open to such a radical suggestion. On the other hand, it is important to remember that it is easier to be stoical and accepting when one is at the top of the food chain, like the emperor Marcus Aurelius. In contrast, if your client can't find a job that pays well enough to keep their family afloat and has difficulty finding good medical care and good childcare, it is not nearly as easy to be accepting.

Other, Possible Between-Session/Self-Help Work

1. Make an appointment with an internist, psychiatrist, or some other health care professional such as a physical therapist.
2. Make an appointment with a lawyer, for example, to get a will written or with a financial advisor or tax accountant.
3. Read:
    David Burns's *Feeling Good*
    Steve Hayes's *Get Out of Your Mind & Into Your Life*

Albert Ellis's *A New Guide to Rational Living*
Martha Davis and her associates' *The Relaxation and Stress Reduction Workbook*
Marsha Linehan's *DBT Skills Training Manual*
Bessel van der Kolk's *The Body Keeps the Score*
Victor Frankl's *Man's Search for Meaning*
Po Bronson's *What Should I Do with My Life?*
Ron Leifer's *Vinegar into Honey*
The Dalai Lama, Desmond Tutu, and D. C. Abrams's *The Book of Joy*
Rollo May's *Love and Will*
Erick Fromm's *The Art of Loving*
Alain de Botton's *How to Think More about Sex*
Jeffrey Schwartz's *Brain Lock: Free Yourself from Obsessive-Compulsive Behavior*
Thich Nhat Hanh's *The Art of Living*

Bibliotherapy may also include the Bible—one of the oldest self-help books in the world—the Koran, the Bhagavad Gita, or Buddhist and Sufi stories, as well as wisdom stories from other cultures and traditions.

1. Watch helpful YouTube videos (e.g., Thich Nhat Hanh).
2. Attend a self-help group like SMART Recovery, AA, Recovery Dharma, LifeRing, Women for Sobriety online or face to face.
3. Volunteer.
4. Dance; take dancing lessons.
5. Bake, cook.
6. Attend a weekend workshop or retreat, for example, at Kripalu, the Omega Institute, the Esalen Institute, and so on.
7. If a client is religious, going to a service or to light a candle or make an offering may help, especially if their religion has been very important to them and they have been ignoring it. But if that is not the case, it is not appropriate as a therapist or counselor to push such an idea.
8. Spending a weekend at a bed and breakfast—away from the everyday environment—may help a couple's relationship more than a therapy session. This is true even if the couple does not have children. Trying to make love in the same environment with all of its stressful cues and triggers simply may not work. Change the environment and many couples find they still love each other.

PART IV

Other Issues

Chapter 17

Self/Selves, Identity/Identities, and Change

Who am I?
What's wrong with me?
Why am I such a failure?
Why is everyone thinking about me?
What should I do?
What have I done?

Most humans trouble themselves with such questions at various times during their lives. A client's sense of self, what they think of themselves and what they have done or not done with their lives, is often the elephant in the room. They have sought out therapy because they are anxious, having trouble with relationships, and/or depressed, but a larger, existential issue may actually be at the core of their problems.

After working for a while with people with addictive and semi-addictive behaviors, I slowly started to realize that I did not know a client who had changed an addictive behavior who had not also wanted to be—and the phrase may not be exactly correct—another type of person. They wanted to be a better partner or father. Or they wanted to be a more successful business-person. Or, if they had been a hard drinking and life-of-the-party kind of person in their 20s, they didn't want to be seen like that in their 30s. They came to accept that they couldn't go on behaving as they had been and be the kind of person they wanted to be going forward. They had to change.

At the end of her very moving video (https://www.nytimes.com/video/health /100000000877082/the-power-of-rescuing-others.html), Linehan says,

> I had this unbelievable experience of God loving me, and I jumped up and ran out and ran to my room. I was standing in my room, and I said—I think out loud—I said, "I love myself." And the minute, the very minute the word "myself" came out of my mouth, I knew I had been completely transformed. Because up to that point, I would have never said that. I would have said, "I love you." Because I had no *sense of self* [emphasis added]. I thought of myself as you. And the minute the word myself came out of my mouth, I knew and I've always known—ever since—I would never, ever cross that line again—to being crazy.

Linehan's religious experience totally transformed her sense of self, and she went on to develop DBT, helping thousands of people by doing so.

IDENTITY/IDENTITIES

How do your clients identify themselves?

How do they think of themselves in terms of class, gender, race, ethnicity, religious affiliation, and even physical and psychological difficulties? Clients who have been diagnosed as "bipolar" or "borderline" often do not like the label or the stigma associated with such diagnoses. How does that contribute to the problems that they want to work on?

My client Claudette identifies herself as a New Yorker. She is also gay, another part of her identity. And she is a mother, which for her is both an identity and a role. But she is very clear that she does not want her identity to be solely tied up with being a mother. She is also a successful businesswoman. She is a good mother; she fulfills that role well. But she prefers to see herself as a businesswoman—who happens to be lesbian—who is also a mother.

Identities have attributes, and some people will like them while others won't. Some people like the directness of New Yorkers. Other people find that quality rude and crude. As Padesky (1989) pointed out many years ago, when a client reports always being worried about what people think of them, what they think of themselves may have to be dealt with first. In an article about using cognitive therapy with lesbian clients, she wrote: "One of the greatest sources of distress for the newly identified lesbian is her own homophobic beliefs. She may tell the therapist that she is concerned only with what others may think. The client may be right that family members and friends will be prejudiced; however, before a lesbian can cope with others' beliefs, she must confront her own" (pp. 147–148).

IDENTITIES, THE SELF, AND A MULTIPLICITY OF SELVES

Although some people say that Buddhism embraces the idea that there is no "self," Thanissaro Bhikku (2014) relates that, in one of the many famous stories about the Buddha, one of his disciples confronts him and asks, "Is there a self?" The Buddha looks away. Answering would have taken the disciple down a wormhole of thinking about self and no-self, all of it a waste of time. The Buddha advised all the monks to avoid getting involved in questions such as "What am I?" "Do I exist?" "Do I not exist?" because they lead to answers like "I have a self" and "I have no self," both of which are a "thicket of views, a writhing of views, a contortion of views" that get in the way of awakening (p. 2).

Westerners definitely think they have a self but most also have some sort of tripartite model in their head. Psychoanalysis borrowed the model with the devil on one shoulder and the angel on the other, calling one the id ("it" in German), the other the superego ("above I" in German), and the third part, the ego ("I" in German) struggling in the middle to manage to live a reasonably non-neurotic life. Transactional analysis, perhaps one of the most popular neo-Freudian models, asserted that everyone was a combination of child, parent, and adult. DBT encourages clients to embrace a different tripartite model of the self: the emotional mind, the rational mind, and the wise mind. DBT-ers try to practice using their wise mind, a balance of the emotional and rational mind, to deal with the vicissitudes of life more effectively. Finally, ACT teaches clients to think of themselves as three selves: the "conceptualized self," the "self as ongoing self awareness," and the "observing self" (Hayes & Smith, 2005, chap. 7).

When I met Ellis, he introduced me to the thinking and writings of Alfred Korzybski, the founder of general semantics. Korzybski forcefully argued that any sentence with the verb *to be* in the middle was inherently faulty: *I am fat. I'm a failure. You're an idiot. Life is unfair.*

Those sentences are grammatically correct, and they seem to make sense, but Korzybski argued that they don't. Your client may think she is fat, but her parents and doctors may think something very different. Your client may have failed at something, but that does not mean they are a failure at everything. Someone in their life may have acted stupidly or unfairly, but that does not make them an idiot. No doubt, at many times, life seems to us to be unfair, but it is not always so.

In essence, it is impossible to evaluate and judge the self or others or life at any moment in time. People may do it, but it is inevitably inaccurate and unstable. Our neurochemistry, how we think and feel, and how we behave changes from minute to minute and from situation to situation. William James suggested that we have a multiplicity of selves. The self that meets the president of Harvard is not the same self that interacts with a daughter or the same self that interacts with a close friend. Sociologists focus on our social identities, that is, which groups we associate ourselves with. Our identity or identities are also affected by how we sense people see us.

Clearly, there are many ways to think of the "self," if one exists at all. Most clients think of themselves in terms of one self and judge that self in many different ways. This may be partly due to our socialization and our genes. People may also see themselves as having a unitary self because, in fact, they are an object. They can and do photograph themselves, often repeatedly. In addition, many people believe in some kind of unitary concept like the soul or transcendent self or higher self. Christianity and Islam teach that at the day of judgment, souls will be judged and sent to heaven or hell. Even Hindus and Buddhists believe something has existed before this current life and will pass on to the next life. Consequently, it is easy and reasonable that people think of their "self" and often evaluate "it." But those evaluations and the thoughts about the evaluations often add to the psychological difficulties that clients are grappling with. Being more mindful of how we think about the self and about identity can help us work more effectively with clients who may have very different conceptualizations about the self and their identity than we do.

"CHARACTER" VERSUS "PERSONALITY"

There is a key difference between character and personality. You can work on and develop grit, resilience, and higher tolerance for frustration and discomfort. In the late 1890s, the focus was on developing character in young people. In *Talks to Teachers and Students* (1900), William James urged educators to help their students cultivate characteristics that young people needed in order to become good citizens and lead healthy, meaningful lives. They included *pugnacity*, which he defined as a "general unwillingness to be beaten by any kind of difficulty . . . and is essential to a spirited and enterprising character" (p. 54), which sounds very much like what we refer to as *resilience*.

At the turn of the 19th century, the focus shifted from "character" to "personality." Personality is fixed, or almost so, although psychoanalysis was supposed to be designed to restructure a patient's personality. Corporations now spend over $500 million giving people tests such as the Myers & Briggs, even though few if any of them have scientific validity. But humans like labels and categories. Labels supposedly help people understand themselves and others.

"BPD," "ego," "id," and "superego," "evil" and "the devil" are all "hypothetical constructs." They cannot be precisely defined or measured. But many people, including clients, like and use terms like these so easily and frequently that they think they are like molecules and germs.

Textbox 17.1. Case—Steve: Can You Be a Cocaine Addict and a Mensch?

Steve, a tough but inherently kind man who worked managing buildings in New York City, had been using cocaine for years. He was in my office because he and his wife wanted to adopt a child, and he wanted to get off cocaine first. He claimed that his wife did not know that he was using, even though his nose was enormously swollen and red. He told her he was very allergic to pollen and so on, and he used only after she went to bed. He needed only about five hours of sleep, so he would use from 10:00 p.m. to 2:00 or 3:00 in the morning.

We worked together for a while, and we started to talk about religious beliefs. He was Jewish but did not practice or believe in religion. Nevertheless, he said, "I want to be a mensch." Those of you who are not from New York may not know that a mensch is a person who tries to do the right thing. Some people may quibble with that definition, but we agreed that we were not talking about trying to be a saint.

We also agreed that in New York at that time, the late 1980s, you could be a cocaine addict (his term) and good lawyer. You could be a cocaine addict and do very well in the fashion industry. And you could be a cocaine addict and very successful in the restaurant business. But you could not be a cocaine addict and a mensch. They were incompatible.

For one year he tried to stop but kept slipping back. He was still working successfully, and his marriage was intact. I finally suggested that he should try some other form of therapy. I gave him referrals to a good outpatient place in the city and to another practitioner. We agreed that if a baseball player keeps hitting poorly, he needs to find a new batting coach. I assured him that another therapist would use a different approach and techniques and have a different sense of humor. It might do the trick.

A year later, I got a call. "Can I come back and work with you, if you promise not to fire me?"

"Of course," I said. "And I didn't fire you."

"Well, it felt like you did, so will you promise not to do it again?"

That was a tricky question.

"I don't like to waste people's time or money. I felt we were wasting your time and money. But I'll be happy to try again. However, I want you to see a psychiatrist I know at the same time. Okay?"

He agreed.

The psychiatrist I suggested was a wonderful woman, very direct and with a great sense of humor, and she definitely helped. In our first meeting, I suggested that he seemed to be dancing around the problem but not really doing what was necessary to change. He told me that in the first meeting with the psychiatrist, she was blunter: "Are you sure you're not just bullshitting yourself?" she had asked him. The combination of my comment and her question, plus another year of getting older and perhaps wiser, did the needful. He stopped and never started again. He told me that, ultimately, he wanted to be a mensch more than a cocaine addict.

But they are not. We can run a test to see if you have COVID. After 50 years of looking for an "addictive personality disorder," there is zero evidence that one exists, but some readers will probably remain convinced that there is such a thing. We have instruments, paper, and pencil tests that supposedly determine if you have a borderline personality disorder, but five personality disorders were so questionable that they almost got completely dropped from the *DSM-5*. A last-minute vote kept them in the book.

In one study (Zanarini et al., 2010), 73% of people who were "diagnosed" with borderline personality disorder (BPD), six years later no longer met the criteria for BPD. That suggests that personality may not be such an enduring construct as some people would like to think. As you may know, Linehan took a very different approach. She believed that people, most often women, who were diagnosed with BPD could learn to regulate their emotions better and behave differently by learning new skills, especially mindfulness skills. It would require at least a year of very hard work, but it was doable.

How is all this relevant for us as therapists and counselors? If you see your client as having a relatively fixed "disorder," for example, a "borderline personality disorder," in your eyes, they may see that you don't think they can change. In contrast, if you think of someone as able to learn how to manage their emotions better, that is very different. Your clients will see that in your eyes, too. (See Research Note, chapter 3, regarding Leake & King, 1977.)

The research is clear, and many people know it personally. It is possible to develop "grit" and "resilience." Carol Dweck (1986, 2015), who almost single-handedly ended the "self-esteem" movement in education and parenting, demonstrated in her research that children who are praised for working hard versus those who are praised for their "brilliance," develop a better "mindset" and do better in school. Students can learn to "work harder." They cannot learn to be more brilliant. She also showed that young people praised as brilliant learn to avoid taking on harder tasks. They might fail and that might diminish their "brilliance" in their parents' or teachers' eyes. Fortunately, students and adults can learn how to stay on task longer and to suffer through discomfort at failing. They can push themselves to be better at math or Spanish or soccer.

INTERSECTIONALITY

According to Singh and colleagues (2021), the term *intersectionality*, "coined by Crenshaw (1989), refers to the connectedness and overlap of different social identities (e.g., race, gender, sexual orientation) related to an individual or group and related to systems of oppression. The theory of intersectionality allows for a broader, contextualized, and more nuanced understanding of individuals' experiences based on their interconnected identities" (p. 956).

Class, racial, culture, ethnicity, sexual/gender, and religious identities may all intersect in unusual and not necessarily stable ways. Clients who are not members of the dominant ethnic or economic class in a country may feel oppressed for a variety of interacting, interdependent reasons, and different clients will no doubt perceive their identities in very different ways.

Textbox 17.2. Dissociative Identities Disorder (DID)

Dissociative identities disorder (DID) is an extremely rare disorder with a long and controversial history. According to the theory, one person may manifest two or more identities at various times. Each identity has its own gender, tone of voice, way of relating to the world, behaviors, and memories and sometimes even blood pressure. One identity is considered the "core identity" and the others are referred to as "alters"; those in favor of accepting all forms of neurodiversity do not think the condition necessarily has to be treated. That is, there is no ethical reason why the alters must be integrated into the core.

It is hypothesized that DID usually develops as the result of severe trauma. It is a way for a person to disassociate or put some distance between what happened and their everyday life. Initially, according to Ian Hacking (1998), it drew the attention of physicians in the late 1880s and 1890s partly because they were anti-Catholic. If they could prove that more than one "person" could inhabit one body, they believed that that would discredit the Catholic notion of a soul. The thinking was that one body could not possibly have two souls.

Enthusiasm for the diagnosis has increased and decreased dramatically over the years and the name itself was changed from multiple personality disorder to DID. Some believe that therapists may inadvertently create signs of the disorder via their own fascination with alters.

WHAT CAN YOU DO?

Clarify the Problem

Perhaps the source of the problem or one of your client's problems involves their identity and the way they think of themselves in life. Since the 1900s, the focus in clinical psychology has been on treating a variety of "disorders," and, more recently, the primary focus, almost obsession, has been on the brain. This type of focus fails to take into account the whole person's reality in the context of their family, culture, job, religion, goals, values, and sense of themselves in time.

Rogers (1951) thought that most of the conflict within people was a result of a discrepancy, sometimes large, between a client's "ideal self" and "real self." He would ask clients to hold their hands out in front of them as if they were going to clap. Next, they were to move them far apart. Then, with one hand representing the ideal self and the other hand the real self, they were to bring their hands together slowly until they felt that they couldn't move them closer without violating reality, the "distance" between their ideal and real self. For Rogers, one object of therapy was to help clients shrink that gap, perhaps reducing it to zero.

Montesano and his associates (2017), in an intriguing research report, suggest that some people may be stuck in therapy (and in life) because they identify themselves as a "good person," a person who "cares for others" and a "sensitive" person. To move forward in their career, in their mind, would require them to change their identity. In their mind, a "successful" businessperson cannot also be a "good," "sensitive" person. Montesano calls this conflict an "implicative dilemma." Moving forward would imply that they were giving up one identity for another, and they do not want to do so. However, they do want to advance in their career. So, they are stuck. And, as a result, often depressed. Without uncovering this conflict in identities, no change may occur.

One of my clients, raised in a very conservative religious family, wanted to leave her religion. In her parents' mind, she would become a "sinner" and burn in hell for eternity. To embrace her new identity, in her mind, she would have to change from being a "good Christian" and a "good daughter" to something very different. Padesky, in the article cited above, reports on working with a client who was grappling with accepting herself as lesbian. Because of her own anti-homosexual beliefs, her client had a very difficult time accepting that new identity.

Provide Unconditional Regard

Providing a place—your office—where clients feel what Rogers labeled "unconditional regard" can also be very healing. In essence, no matter what clients report, you treat them with respect. This does not mean you respect all of their behavior. What you hear you may not respect for a variety of reasons. But you can still treat them with respect. Your regard remains constant. They are humans who are trying to accept aspects of themselves, others, and their world, and, at the same time, in some ways, change. A safe place—your office—and a non-judgmental person listening carefully and empathetically—you—will help the healing process.

A good, safe working relationship has to be developed, and that may take time. Then the reality of identifying with being gay or non-white or poor or Muslim or Asian or female or transgender or with a physical or psychological disability or some combination may be addressed. Lefevor and his associates (2022) emphasize the importance of making clear to clients that our "only stake in our clients' process is their self-understanding and mental health" (p. 490).

Process Inequity, Injustice, Racism, and Classism

I was fortunate in the 1970s to be working on the campus with women who worked for the newly founded Feminist Press. They introduced me to feminist theory and feminist therapy and the writing and thinking of people like Dr. Florence Howe, the press's founder, Dr. Laura Brown (2004), and Andrea Dworkin. The movements they were involved in affected my thinking; they encouraged discussion of ideas that were generally not honored in therapy. CBT helps clients analyze and process thoughts and beliefs to see to what extent they are rational or irrational, helpful or unhelpful. But, as Lyrica Fils-Aimé (2021) points out, whether a thought or belief is "irrational" or "unhelpful" will depend on the context. If your client has been marginalized or treated badly or unfairly based on an aspect of their identity, what they are thinking—*Everybody is looking at me. I could get killed here.*—may not be irrational or unhelpful. It may keep them alive. She writes: "We as therapists should validate the negative thoughts, because survival is one reason that one may have developed such thinking, and it may be protective" (n.p.).

Moreover, your client may be very good at what they do, but race, class, gender, or some other factor may be preventing them from moving up in their career. Not only can you validate the injustice of this reality, but you can also help a client learn to develop their inner criteria (see below) and evaluate their behavior on their own terms. As a result, they may feel better about themselves although not necessarily about the world.

For years, at the institute, the receptionist was a wonderful Black woman named Shari. One day, for the first time ever, she called in saying that she didn't feel well. Over the next few days, she didn't come to work. Shari had never been sick, but she went to the emergency room of her local hospital twice and was sent home twice. No one asked her about her mother's medical history. Her mother had died of a heart attack at age 52. Two days later Shari died, at home, of a silent heart attack, at age 52. The research is clear. Had she been male and white, she probably would have received better care. What's the point? When a white, male client says and believes strongly, *People are against me*, he may be thinking irrationally, and that kind of thinking will create problems for him. In contrast, when someone from a marginalized group thinks that way, that may not be irrational or problematic.

Encourage a Pluralistic Perspective

I think most people would agree that if they are a therapist or a lawyer that this is part of their identity. It is one way that other people think of them and that they think of themselves. James Clear, the author of *Atomic Habits* (2018), one of the most popular books on changing habits, has suggested that anything you do repeatedly can be seen as part of the person you are. If you often bake bread, you are a baker, and that is part of who you are. You are not a professional baker, but you are one who bakes, presumably fairly often. If you go skiing every season, you are a skier, but not necessarily a snowboarder.

I was working once with Tom, a litigator at a medium-sized law firm in New York. He often felt depressed and very anxious. He was not always as good a father as he wanted to be. If something was a problem at his firm, he would get very anxious: he was not as good a lawyer, partner, leader as he thought he should be. I asked him to make a list of all his "identities" or "roles" or "things you do a lot or like to do, like skiing."

Then I asked him to put a number next to each of these "identities." Between 0 and 10, how good a lawyer, father, photographer, neighbor did he think he was? Next, I asked him how much he wanted to be a good lawyer, father, photographer, neighbor, and so on and to put a number, 0–10, next to the first number.

When he came to the next session, he had printed out his list, and handed it to me:

1. Lawyer, 8/10
2. Teacher, 7/10
3. Photographer, 6/9
4. Husband, 9/10
5. Father, 8/10
6. Brother, 8/8
7. Brother-in-law, 7/7
8. Uncle, 8/8
9. Cousin, 7/7
10. Friend, 8/9
11. Neighbor, 8/8
12. Cook, 10/10
13. Bicyclist, 7/7
14. Skier, 7/8
15. Hiker, 9/9
16. Leader in my firm, 8/9
17. Partner in my firm, 8/9

As you can see, he thought he is an 8 as a lawyer, but he wants to be a 10. As a neighbor, he is an 8, and that is good enough. He is content with being an 8.

I sat for a while and then looked up, and as gently as I could, asked, "What about 'loser'?"

We sat quietly for a while.

"I know sometimes you call yourself a 'loser' and a 'failure,'" I added.

Again, we sat for a while.

"Well, looking at this list, I guess I'm not such a 'loser,'" he said. "But these are just roles and things I do, like ski."

"I'm not sure you're correct," I said. "The term *loser* is a global, obscure, negative rating of our entirety. Based on what you've told me, most of your friends see you as a good father and your lawyer friends probably see you as a good lawyer."

"Yes," he said quietly.

Slowly, Tom began to realize that he played many roles and tried to "be" many different types of people. If he wasn't doing so well as a lawyer one day, he did not have to let his "poor lawyering" define his entirety—if he was, in fact, doing poor lawyering, always questionable, especially in someone like Tom. He was not defined by one activity or set of behaviors. His continual ruminating over questions like "Who am I?" with its negative corollaries, "I'm a failure. I'm useless and worthless" gradually receded into the background.

Clear (2018) makes a distinction between outcome-based habits and identity-based habits, that is, habits that are aimed at what you want to accomplish and those that are focused on the person you want to become. He also argues, "The more deeply a thought or action is tied to your identity, the more difficult it is to change. It can feel comfortable to believe what your culture believes (group identity) or to do what upholds your self image (personal identity), even if it's wrong. The biggest barrier to positive change at any level—individual, team, society—is identity conflict" (p. 35). This is very similar to what the research by Montesano and his associates (2017) suggests.

As I noted earlier, in 2010, I ran into the work of Dr. Robert West. West and Brown (2013) hypothesize that wanting to change one's identity from being a "smoker" to a "nonsmoker" may affect not just the "wants" part of one's motivational system but also the planning and evaluation parts. As a result, an intervention that highlights the discrepancy between, in this case, the smoker and the potential nonsmoker may be uniquely effective, something that MI emphasizes.

For most clients, it may be better to focus on what kinds of person they want to be, that is, to think in terms of the plural, not the singular. They can try to be a good Christian or a mensch, but ultimately, that will involve trying to be multiple types of people, that is, a good mother, lawyer, sister, friend, neighbor, and so on.

To Increase "Self-Confidence," Focus on Behaviors

Some clients want to have more self-confidence, with an emphasis on the "self." No doubt, we meet and interact with people who seem, and may well be, confident about everything they do. But your client may not be wired up like that. I suggest an alternative to "*self*-confidence," one focused on behaviors. For example, it may work better to focus on becoming a more confident driver or a more confident teacher or salesperson or a more confident cook than on overall self-confidence.

Confidence is a combination of competence and a willingness to accept that something might go wrong, maybe very wrong. Clients can develop more competence by practicing. In contrast, there is not much a client can do to improve their "self." And they can work—perhaps with you, if they wish to—to accept that something may go very wrong.

However, even evaluating a behavior can be tricky. The evaluation may vary by person and time. Someone may have thought your client did a very good job making a presentation and another person may think otherwise. Someone may think that the bread your client baked is fantastic while another person may not find it so. That is when working with a client to develop their own "inner criteria" may be very helpful.

Provide an Alternative: Inner Criteria

Unfortunately, some clients are like puppets with the strings to their emotional life held by their boss, a partner or spouse, a parent, a sibling, or a peer. Their opinion of themselves totally hinges on what someone else thinks. If their boss is happy with their performance, they're happy. If not, they're miserable. The same may be true with friends and their partner. Alternatively, if they evaluate their behavior based on their own inner criteria, they will feel and do better over time.

Someone who cooks good pasta sauce has their own idea about what makes a good sauce, that is, their own inner criteria. Other people may not agree with them, but they know what they think. Without being aware of it, clients probably have already developed their own inner criteria for many things in their life—clothes, food, cars, jobs, and persons.

Initially, find something that your client is good at. How do they know they're good at it? What are their criteria? Subsequently, find something that they would like to be good at, for example, talking to a boss or giving a presentation. If they want to be more confident in making presentations, what do they need to do well? How would they know they had given a good presentation? What are their own criteria? Whether or not their boss liked it is, for the purpose of this exercise, totally irrelevant. What do *they* think? How good was it? What/how could they have done better? That is what needs to be looked at when one is developing one's inner criteria.

Managing the Committee's Inner Critics

How and in what ways does one or more members of your client's "committee" negatively rate their selves, their behavior, other people, and the world? What part of their identity or identities does their committee attack? Does an inner critic tend to rate their entire self negatively whenever they make a mistake?

All people learn all kinds of things sitting in their high chairs observing the world and trying to figure it out. Later they absorb all sorts of "rules" and "shoulds" from their parents and other family members, their peers, and the media. Those rules and shoulds and should-nots help them survive. At about age 12, they start to add their own shoulds: *I shouldn't have to wear cheap sneakers when everyone else has really good ones. My brother shouldn't get to stay out later than I can.* A thousand shoulds, a "tyranny of the should[s]," as Horney put it (1950, pp. 64–65).

Gradually, clients can be helped to become more aware of their "shoulds" and to speak more kindly to themselves about themselves and their behaviors. At times, their peers and the media in all of its myriad forms may overwhelm them, and that is when a good therapist or counselor may be critically important in helping them learn to navigate their complex world and to embrace their identities and idiosyncrasies.

Textbox 17.3. Case—Arianna: Doing It My Way

Years ago, I wanted to help a client, Arianna, prepare for a business presentation. She was very anxious about doing it. In the past, she had always hated presentations, and she avoided them as much as possible. In a sense, she had good reason to be anxious. She had not practiced making presentations very often, and, as a result, she had not developed much competence in making them.

But Arianna had decided that she wanted to become the first Latina vice president in the company, and that would require making many more presentations and doing so with confidence.

She feared her boss's assessment, because she felt he would be judging her as woman and a non-white woman, at that. Given that the company did not have many female vice presidents, let alone non-white vice presidents, that was probably not irrational.

I suggested that judging her performance on the basis of her own criteria, independent of what her boss might think, would help. That was really all that she could control. I knew she liked to do well, and this would give her an opportunity to hone an important skill which she was lacking. After the presentation, she could take some time to "grade" her presentation and to reflect on its good and not-so-good points and learn from the experience.

We made a list of the characteristics of a good presentation: well organized, tells a story, announces at the beginning the objective of the presentation, sums up the points at the end, starts with a pause and a friendly greeting to the audience and key people in the audience, ends with a thank you to everyone, and especially to her boss for the opportunity to make the presentation. Ideally, her voice would be calm, and she would sound confident and fully prepared.

We also talked about how she might not do everything she had set out to do in the way that she wanted to do it. How would she interpret that? How could she interpret that instead? What could she do to best respond to that situation?

Over the next week Arianna did seven things to increase the probability that she would make a good presentation: She wrote out what she wanted to say. She practiced it in front of a mirror. She practiced it in front of her roommate. She practiced it at the level of imagery, working on letting go of unhelpful thoughts like *This HAS to go well or I'm finished.* She went to the gym the day before her presentation. She drank only a very little coffee that morning. And as she sat waiting to be asked to make her presentation, she used a guided imagery exercise to get her ready to step up to the podium, ready to go.

Afterward, she took some time to reflect on the experience and to give the presentation—not herself—a "grade." She thought it went quite well: 85. Better than she expected. But there were some things she thought that she could have done even better.

It turned out that her boss also thought she had done a good job. She was pleased, very pleased that he liked it. But she stuck to her own rating. She had worked on developing her own criteria, aware that if she only felt good when her boss liked what she did, she would be like a puppet, with her emotional life at the mercy of her boss's likes and dislikes and other idiosyncrasies. The presentation had gone well. She had done an 85. And she could work on getting better at it if she wanted to.

Some Questioning Is Harmful

As noted in chapter 14, some questions may be harmful. When a client says in a frustrated tone, *"I don't even know who I am. Who am I?"* I may suggest that that is a "trap question." As Korzybski (1958) asserted, it sounds sensible and is grammatically correct, but it is unanswerable. At least, there is no short answer. The long answer may be that they are a New Yorker, a therapist, a father, a cook, a fisherman, and so forth. But some form of self-criticism and self-pity often lies hidden underneath these sorts of questions, a feeling that whoever or whatever they are is inadequate. They don't measure up.

As I noted in chapter 7, humans rate everything all of the time including themselves and their actions, feelings, and thoughts. Questions like *Who am I?* are inherently difficult if not impossible to answer. Moreover, such questions often contribute to a client feeling helpless, hopeless, and trapped. Helping them become more aware of what is actually going on—that they are actually criticizing themselves in the form of questions—and helping them stop such behavior may significantly help them over the long run.

Help Your Client Manage Unconscious Bias

Without rating we could not make judgments about how to talk to a stranger, who to try to cultivate as a friend, or who to hire and fire. Unfortunately, our rating may be based on a very few attributes. Research suggests that many interviewers have decided about a job applicant in the first few minutes. However, that kind of thinking often helps continue racism, classism, and other chronic problems in our society.

David F. George (2021) points out in his book *Unconscious Bias,*

> The human brain automatically feels at ease when we interact with people we think and look alike, or act similarly. That was used as a survival trick in the savannah and is still applicable today. Our brain creates shortcuts to handle the important information it processes. These shortcuts cause us to make quick and snappy decisions about who or what we prefer over others. It is these automatic preferences that we refer to as biases. And the fact that our brain does it without awareness is what makes it unconscious. (p. 5)

Because people are often not conscious of their biases, a nonjudgmental, gentle approach may be even more important when working on this aspect of a problem.

Chapter 18

Integrating Coaching

Many traditional psychotherapists feel that coaching and therapy cannot coexist. In contrast, modern integrative therapists recognize that people often can be helped by direct suggestions. Empathic, psychodynamically informed "active listening" is sometimes not sufficient if one wants therapy and counseling to be effective.

The supposed conflict between "coaching" and "therapy/counseling" may stem from the Freudian and neo-Freudian influenced training of many traditional therapists. As I have discussed earlier (see chapter 2), their underlying theories are predicated on the idea that the source of psychological disturbance is buried deep in the unconscious and cannot be directly addressed. Insight into the roots of the problem can only be gained by watching for clues in dreams, slips of the tongue, transference, countertransference, and so on. It is a slow, arduous process. Traditional therapy is also based on the idea that people who come to therapy are "damaged" and need to be fixed or healed. And most traditional therapy was not and is not collaborative.

Those who practice a more client-centered, solution-focused approach, in contrast, strongly believe in the innate health of the people they work with. They often refuse to call them "patients." They are not sick. Hence, they call them "clients." They also believe that clients are generally aware of their difficulties and can state what they want to work on. However, many client-centered therapists also very strongly believe in letting people find their own way. That is, they are, like Rogers, very nondirective. This, of course, is not true of coaches. Coaching is explicitly directive.

Most traditional therapists and counselors still believe that the answers to problems reside in the past and some sort of deep work is necessary. No doubt, many people who wind up in therapy are there because of significant negative events in their childhood, including trauma due to sexual, emotional, and physical abuse. Ignoring such childhood events would be counterproductive and probably unethical. However, as I have suggested throughout this book, many other factors may play a role, including conditioning and neurochemistry, for which "deep" therapy, on its own, is ineffective.

In elementary schools, some teachers and students prefer the "discovery method." Children are encouraged to discover aspects of their world, in terms of science, mathematics, literature, and art. Other teachers and students prefer a more direct, didactive approach. The teachers teach their students what they think their students should learn. Some students do better with such an approach. In many ways, traditional therapy follows the discovery method. Many therapists still essentially let the client talk. Eventually what needs to be talked about will be talked about and "processed" and the client will get better. Modern integrated counseling and psychotherapy advocates for a mixed, combined approach, some time spent in nondirective, discovery activities and some on building new skills in a more didactic manner.

Even if, with some clients, the roots of some problems are buried and will take time to uncover and to process, it still makes sense to help people to learn how to better handle the emotional ups and downs that are currently impeding their ability to fulfill their goals. It will help if they develop more resilience, better distress tolerance, mindfulness and acceptance, and compassion for themselves and others. In that case, therapy and coaching go naturally together. DBT, for example, explicitly includes phone coaching for this purpose.

Similarly, some form of coaching can play a significant role even if your client and/or you think that the problem may be the result of a neurochemical imbalance. Traditionally, to fix that problem meant following the doctor's orders and swallowing a pill. Fortunately, we now know that there are many other ways to change neurochemistry, including changing the way a client thinks about things, meditation, better sleep hygiene, better eating habits, and more physical movement. All may be helped along by direct teaching and coaching.

Modern integrative therapy has many similarities with coaching and some distinct differences.

Similarities:

1. In both coaching and therapy, the client wants to change.
2. Both are focused on goals.
3. Both are active, directive.
4. Both use a combination of techniques to help their clients.
5. Between-session work may be as significant as, if not more significant than, what occurs in a session.
6. Both coaches and modern therapists know ways to help their clients, but their relationship is more collaborative than top-down.

Differences:

1. Coaches who are not already trained counselors or therapists will not know how to work on the roots of some of the problems that may impede progress. For example, someone's social anxiety and/or depression may prevent them from doing what a coach suggests. Or issues with authority may stem from childhood problems with an overbearing parent and may make improving a relationship with a boss impossible. Consequently, people who turn to a modern therapist will do better when those issues are addressed, in addition to being coached as they develop new skills to handle issues, such as low distress tolerance or emotional self-regulation.
2. If a company hires a coach to help one of its employees, the coach probably will be expected to report back to the employer (the company) in terms of how successful or unsuccessful the coaching has been. Hence, someone who goes to a coach cannot count on confidentiality. Some people would argue, perhaps correctly, that when insurance companies get involved, one can't be sure a diagnosis (or diagnoses) will be kept confidential either. That may be true, but it is expected that what you say to a counselor or therapist is totally confidential, with a very few exceptions. That may not be the case with a coach, so clients may not divulge important information.
3. To date, coaching is not regulated in any state in the United States, and one doesn't have to have any training to open a coaching practice. That concerns those who fear that some people will be harmed by going to a coach who isn't trained to handle serious psychological difficulties. In addition, some coaches may be overconfident in their ability to

treat emotional and behavior problems. The research of Kraus and his associates (2011) strongly suggests that no therapist or counselor is good at everything. There is little reason to think coaches are any different.

4. Coaches are not held to the same legal requirements regarding dual relationships, as is true for most therapists and counselors.
5. On the plus side, going to a coach does not have any stigma attached to it. In fact, many people boast that they have a coach and volunteer their name.
6. Finally, insurance companies generally don't pay for coaching because insurance pays for treatments for illnesses. A diagnostic code is required for insurance reimbursement.
7. Most coaches do not have "supervisors." No matter what term you use, supervisor or consultant, it is absolutely essential to have an experienced person who you can count on to help you when you have concerns about what is happening with a client. Most coaches do not have such a person.

WHAT CAN YOU DO?

Those of us who have advanced degrees in counseling, social work, and clinical psychology are perhaps the best trained to help people with the complex problems of life. Dentists study and focus on teeth, cardiologists on the heart, and so forth. We study and continue to study how people grapple with what life throws at them. We look at the whole person within their social and professional contexts.

Slow Discussions for Couples

Teaching couples this technique helps them discuss how they feel about crucial issues in their relationship in a slower, calmer manner. The rules are quite simple, but not necessarily easy to follow, so coaching in session helps.

1. Person A picks a topic/problem and talks about it *for a brief period of time.*
2. When they are finished, they say, "I'm finished."
3. Person B may not say anything while A is talking, even when B has a strong urge to interrupt and rebut what they're hearing. They may not talk until they hear A say, "I'm finished."
4. When A says, "I'm finished," B should take a moment and figure out how they feel about what they've heard. Feelings are generally one word: hurt, sad, hopeful, angry, alone, anxious, furious, bereft. B starts their response with a feeling word or several feeling words. For example, "I feel really sad when I hear what you said." or "I feel very angry and betrayed." Then B can talk about what they think. While they are talking, A may not interrupt until they hear B say, "I'm finished."
5. Then A should sit for a moment to figure out how they feel, and then respond with one or more feeling words.
6. They then can explain why and talk until they say, "I'm finished."

Each person is encouraged to talk briefly and to not drag into the conversation everything that they may feel hurt or angry about from the past. When I think it is appropriate, I may ask them to limit what they talk about to the past two weeks.

The "feeling" part of this exercise is the most difficult for clients and they often benefit from coaching. It is common for the second person to say, "I think that it's really unfair for you to say . . . " This is a thought, an opinion, not a feeling.

Starting a response by telling their partner how they feel helps them communicate from their "heart," not their "head." Including the "I'm finished" part slows down the whole conversation. The person talking knows that the other person will not interrupt until they say, "I'm finished." Many arguments devolve into a shouting match. No one has a chance to stop and think about how they feel. They just want to get in the next shot.

"A" may start about a problem and then go on and on about everything they are upset about. Coaching them to pick one thing and to talk only a few minutes, two or three, about that helps. "B" can't figure out how they feel about multiple problems. Coaching a couple how to use this technique can help them learn to discuss very difficult issues at home in a slower, more compassionate manner.

Caution: What You Should NOT Try to Do

Giving advice for a relationship problem is always a bad idea. As William James pointed out, relationships are mysterious and very difficult, if not impossible, to understand: "Every Jack sees in his own particular Jill charms and perfections to the enchantment of which we stolid onlookers are stone-cold. And which has the superior view of the absolute truth, we or he?" (James, 1900, p. 179). We may think we know what is going on in a marriage, but how much do we really know about what happens in the kitchen or the bedroom? What is it that attracts one person to another? From a scientific, research point of view, we have practically no idea. In addition, do you really want someone angrily sitting in your office, yelling, "You told me to break up with Alice!" or "You told me to tell Ramon how I felt!" You may not think that is what you did, but that is the way your advice was taken.

Assertiveness Training and Role-Playing

If a client is anxious about going on an interview or talking to a boss or a spouse or parent, role-playing and reverse role-playing work very effectively to help them become more adept at asking a boss for a raise, defending themselves in a fight with an argumentative spouse, and setting boundaries.

At first, they may benefit from switching roles. For example, they take the role of a boss, and you take their place, demonstrating how and what they might say. Or they take the role of an angry, hypercritical parent, and you take their role.

Role-playing is a very powerful therapeutic technique, but, unfortunately, many counselors and therapists never suggest or use it. Chairwork, a related technique, can also be very powerful.

Coaching and the ABC Technique

The ABC technique is a very popular self-help tool, but it is not easy to learn. Coaching clients on how to do an ABC in your office will help. Having them do one or more between sessions and then going over them in the next session will not only give you considerable insight into how they are thinking but will also make clear what they do and don't understand about how to do an ABC.

Executive Coaching

As you may know, some people combine their therapy and counseling work with executive coaching. If you have had experience at the executive level in corporate settings, NGO offices, or some other form of business before you became a counselor or therapist, this may make sense. You know what those environments are like and may have become adept at office politics. Developing two professions, one to do executive coaching and one to do counseling and therapy, can work very well. However, if you have not had fairly extensive executive-level work experience, it may not be ethical to include executive coaching in your practice.

Life Coaching

Everybody has lived, so unlike executive coaching, I assume everyone may be able to do life coaching. There are now many certification programs available. Is it ethical to give advice solely based on your life and not take any kind of training? Maybe it is. That is for you to decide. By the time you read this, your state or country may have passed laws regulating coaching and, as a result, training may be required before you can start a coaching business.

Chapter 19

Medications: Are They Right for Your Client?

No culture has ever before been so inundated with medications. Most of us start giving our babies medications very, very early in life, including baby forms of aspirin, ibuprofen, and antihistamines. When they are young, if they don't feel well, they are usually given a pill, maybe more than one. They are normalized to taking pills to solve their problems. This is truly not the era that your grandparents or even parents grew up in. Currently, one in five Americans is taking a legally prescribed medication for their mental health, up from one in six 10 years ago. However, almost all medications have side effects, some very subtle but some severe. We also know practically nothing about how they interact within the human body. Most pain and antianxiety medications calm and slow down the entire body, including the gut. As a result, many people experience constipation and take other medications to treat that. How the combination affects the flora and fauna of the gut is little known, but we do know that the microbiota of the gut affects how people feel and behave (Bercik et al., 2011; Tengeler et al., 2020; Zheng et al., 2016).

Fifty years ago, advertising of medications on the television was illegal. Now almost every show contains an ad for a new medication for a new disease. When people feel some kind of "bad," they now reach for a pill. This is unfortunate because there are many other ways to change one's neurochemistry. In addition, once a client has swallowed a pill (or two or three), there is really no way of predicting how that pill (or pills) will affect their physiology or psychology. Women prescribed some antidepressants or antipsychotics will almost certainly gain 50 pounds. That definitely will not help them feel better about themselves or their lives. If they are prescribed those medications because they are at risk of committing suicide, then keeping them alive at the cost of gaining significant weight is understandable. But often that is not the case. They are depressed but not suicidal.

Each individual reacts to different chemicals differently. The pharmaceutical companies downplay this fact. For headaches, some people rely on Advil or Motrin (that is, some type of over-the-counter nonsteroidal anti-inflammatory drug) while others swear by Tylenol (acetaminophen). The effects on different individual neurochemical systems is not imaginary. They are real. Similarly, a particular psychotropic medication may help one person but not another.

Critics often say the medications are only slightly better or no better than a placebo. But whatever happens in a "placebo study" should be examined more carefully by researchers rather than just being dismissed, as Dr. Ted Kaptchuk persuasively points out (in Leopold, 2021). Psychological researchers and neuroscientists could do well to study what actually is happening in an individual due to a "placebo effect."

However, people who have a family member with a psychological illness are fortunate today. No one is living in a dreadful "insane asylum" of years past. No one is in a straitjacket. SSRIs and other medications may be being used by too many people who could get by without them, but the lives of people with serious mental health issues have been completely changed. They are sometimes working and sometimes even extremely successful.

Therapists who take an either-or approach—either talk therapy or medication—may be practicing unethically. They are not trying to help their client in the best way possible. The science of psychotherapy and psychiatry is so young that we really don't know what will work with a specific individual patient and when. We must try a variety and a combination of approaches. Our client will tell us, as best they can, what works for them and what does not.

A medical analogy may help your client make the decision as to whether to add medication. Colds are caused by viruses, and antibiotics won't help. Rest and liquids, such as a good bowl of homemade soup, are the normal "treatment." When a cold turns into pneumonia, however, it is wise to go to a doctor and get a prescription for an antibiotic. Pneumonia may be caused by a bacteriological infection. Without adding an antibiotic to their treatment, they may become seriously ill and possibly die.

In some states, for example, New York, it is not legal for me, a psychologist, to discuss medications with my clients. However, I can explore with them how they feel about medications and what they or a family member may want them to do. What are their beliefs about medications? They may think *I can't get better without medications. I must find a medication that works to get better.* Or, conversely, *Medications won't help. I need to fix this problem on my own without medications.*

Should you encourage your client to combine medications with psychotherapy? This is a difficult question. Some medications may do harm (Angell, 2011a, 2011b), and many appear very difficult to get off (Carey & Gebeloff, 2018; Cosci & Chouinard, 2020; Moncrieff, 2006). On the other hand, some medications may help your client live a much better, happier life. If we are genuinely trying to practice client-centered psychotherapy, we must respect that each client will have to figure out for themselves what works best, talk therapy, medication, or some combination. About half of my clients are on some type of psychotropic medication.

The Pluses and Minuses of Medications

The Pluses: When diagnoses are added to the *DSM*, disorders that may not have been covered in the past become eligible for insurance reimbursements. Many parents were relieved and delighted when what is now called ADHD was added to the *DSM* in 1968. (For readers curious about how the ADHD diagnosis has evolved over the past 50 years, see Epstein & Loren, 2013.)

The Minuses: Some people argue that when the first ADHD diagnosis, hyperkinetic reaction of childhood, and subsequent diagnoses were added, millions of children began to be medicated for what is often just a normal aspect of childhood development. It is true that once a new diagnosis is included in the *DSM*, multiple new medications begin to be marketed, often directly to the public on television. Watters (2010) asserts that pharmaceutical companies and psychiatrists often on their payroll have created markets and enormous profits around the world for disorders that many people previously did not think existed in their cultures. And it is now generally acknowledged that millions of people taking antidepressants might be better served by some form of talk therapy (Boren et al., 2009; DeRubeis et al, 2008).

Considering that we now know that some medications can cause harm and some result in dependency, we need to be cautious about suggesting that a client try medication. On the other hand, at times, when a new client is complaining of psychotic symptoms or looks extremely unhealthy, I may decline to work with them unless and until they consult a psychiatrist or other form of physician.

If a client is ambivalent about going to a psychiatrist, I remind them that a psychiatrist almost always has to give them a prescription. Imagine what might happen if a client consulted with a psychiatrist, and they did not prescribe anything, and then the client committed suicide. But I point out that they can decide to fill the prescription or not. It is up to them. They can fill the prescription and put the medication in their bedside table drawer. I may tell them the story about a client that I recommended see a psychiatrist. I sensed that she was close to having what used to be called a nervous breakdown and now, depending on the symptoms, may be diagnosed as a psychotic break. As it turned out, her condition worsened significantly over the weekend. She called her psychiatrist asking whether she should go to the hospital. He urged her to start the medications which, thankfully, she had on hand, and she did and avoided a hospital stay.

WHAT CAN YOU DO?

Psychiatrist or Internist?

Ultimately, if you're new to the profession, depending on where you work, you may feel forced to decide: Do you want to work primarily like a medical doctor, diagnose your patients, and then try to cure them of their illness? Or, like Rogers (1951), do you want to refer to most of the people who come to see you as "clients," not "patients," because you don't think they're sick. Most readers will wind up with a combined approach. Some clients (or patients) will take medications and definitely benefit from them. Others, who probably could do well without medications, will take them. Some clients who might do much better on medications will refuse to even entertain the idea.

I prefer that my clients see a psychiatrist, not their internist. Psychiatrists focus their entire professional life on medications and have much more experience with how they affect different patients and much more familiarity with the possible side effects. An internist simply does not have enough time to keep up with the ever-expanding number of drugs available. But it is sometimes better if a client sees someone, perhaps their internist, rather than no one at all.

Help Your Client Find the Right Psychiatrist/Psychopharmacologist

A good psychiatrist has been around for a while and has developed a sense of what might be going on, mostly from observing and listening to patients. They will also find out what is going on in a patient's life and perhaps also take into account the patient's culture, socioeconomic class, and even religion. Then, the psychiatrist looks into what they know about various medications and suggests what they think may work best. And after a month or so, if the patient is not doing better, they will suggest trying something different or perhaps a combination of medications. Medications can be a godsend, but psychiatrists cannot yet determine precisely which one might help a particular individual.

Psychiatrists also have to respond to the fact that many medications lose their effectiveness over time. For example, Depakote, a medication for bipolar disorder, sometimes stops helping after only six months in some patients. In addition, many medications have unpleasant and sometimes unacceptable side effects.

It is very helpful to have a good psychiatrist to work with. They can provide you with a different perspective on a patient. Unfortunately, it is not always easy to find a good psychiatrist. What makes for a good psychiatrist? First, they must be kind. This is especially true for a client who has great difficulty managing their thinking, feelings, and behaviors. They may only have friends who also have similar difficulties and, as a result, are not very good at being a friend. Most people avoid them altogether. If they feel "rejected," they may not be being irrational or delusional. It is happening to them. If they reach out to psychiatrists in a frantic manner, even psychiatrists may begin to "reject" them, too. They need to find someone who is compassionate, understanding, and patient.

If your client has been seriously depressed before, they cannot fool themselves into thinking that it will end in two or three days. It will endure. Consequently, some clients may turn to alcohol, a very fast-acting antidepressant, or something else like cocaine. The grinding depression will lift in five minutes. Your patient will feel better. Of course, those wonderful results will not last for long. And with bipolar individuals, they may become even more unstable. But who can blame them for trying to help themselves feel better, if only for a short time?

Unfortunately, psychiatrists may not respond in such a compassionate manner to such behavior. They may suddenly refuse to see your client "until they deal with their substance abuse problem." This completely ignores the fact that the client's mental illness that the psychiatrist is treating may be linked to alcohol misuse. You need to try to find a patient, kind psychiatrist who will work with clients with complex, overlapping problems. It is not always easy.

Overutilized Medications

As the Buddha pointed out more than 2,500 years ago, everyone suffers at least some time in their lives. Almost everyone wishes for life to be different and almost everyone suffers sorrow, sadness, aggravation, and frustration at times during almost every day. It is not surprising that antidepressant, antianxiety, and ADHD medications are sometimes taken in an attempt to cope with the difficulties of everyday life and the resulting negative affect.

Unfortunately, some people suffer more than others. Perhaps because of trauma, especially chronic, long-term trauma, or because of genetic predispositions that are very little understood, some people's neurotransmitters do not work as well. It is not surprising that they may be tempted to overuse various chemicals and even various activities, such as gambling, video gaming, and watching porn, all of which increase dopamine and make many people feel better.

Reportedly, the atypical antipsychotics (AAPs) introduced in the 1990s and designed for the treatment of schizophrenia are now widely prescribed to elderly people with dementia and to children and adolescents, despite the fact that they are not FDA approved for young people (Haw & Stubbs, 2007; Meng et al., 2022; Spielmans, 2015). These are powerful drugs and according to one study, "AAPs are associated to different extents, with weight gain, metabolic syndrome (MetS), and nonalcoholic fatty liver disease (NAFLD)" (Xu & Zhuang, 2019, p. 2087). Not only that but, according to the same study, those problems are not easy to diagnose and the kind of blood testing that should be done is not being done. And, as we know, thousands of people were prescribed pills for pain and now have turned to less expensive street drugs often laced with fentanyl to treat the pain and their addiction caused by the original pills.

Why is this happening? Of course, part of the answer lies in the fact that doctors are being marketed to by well-paid, hired "experts" and often lied to about the possible negative side effects of new medications. (See the video series *Dopesick* for a dramatic depiction of the genesis of the opioid epidemic.) However, most psychiatrists and psychopharmacologists are working very hard to be helpful. They want a patient to be able to go to school or their job.

They don't want their patients to wreck their most important relationships or, worst-case scenario, to commit suicide. At the same time, clients—and parents of children—may be equally desperate to find something to resolve a frightening problem. No one really knows how a medication may help and very little or nothing about how one may interact with several others, but when a life is at risk, taking one more pill does not seem like such a dreadful idea. Unfortunately, as is becoming increasingly evident, for many people, that pathway does not lead to long-term recovery. Combining the medication with some form of talk therapy, mindfulness work, exercise, and other activities is usually necessary.

Underutilized Medications

There are also medications that are underutilized. Again, marketing—in this case, the lack of marketing—is the problem. In our modern world, if something is not advertised, it barely exists. Many of these medications are useful for managing risky health behaviors, such as overdrinking, overeating, smoking, and opioid misuse.

Naltrexone was ballyhooed as the "cure" for alcoholism in the 1990s, ignoring the fact that many people who have problems with overdrinking do not want to be "cured." As is true of most humans, they like altered states of consciousness. But while taking naltrexone, it is very unlikely that they will make a fool out of themselves at a business party or a wedding, a definite plus. But they will not get the buzz or the feeling numb that they may seek.

A person who takes Antabuse will vomit if they drink alcohol. That usually eliminates the struggle that occurs for many people who have problems with alcohol around 5:00 p.m.: *Should I have a drink? No, not tonight.* Then later: *I can't stand the way I feel right now. Yes, I can. This is stupid. No, it's not stupid. I'm just going to eventually have a drink. I can wait one day. No, I can't.* Often these types of inner arguments lead to drinking, but not if one is taking Antabuse. Antabuse provides people some days when there is no inner conflict and helps them figure out how to live—and maybe even enjoy life—without alcohol. This is true even for clients who stop taking Antabuse on Thursday so that they can drink on Friday or Saturday. They have some days when they are not tortured with conflicting thoughts, giving them an opportunity to experience an alcohol-free day or evening.

Methadone has been used for years to help people combat their addiction to heroin, but to take it, people had to line up, usually at a door in the back of the hospital, at 8:00 a.m. with a lot of other people, some homeless, some mentally ill, and some selling methadone and other drugs. Consequently, the vast majority of people who get hooked on heroin avoid using methadone. And if they decide to go through the humiliation of standing in line, they still can't travel or go on vacation. The arrival of suboxone on the market was a godsend. For the first time, people could go to a doctor's office and get a prescription and then go to their pharmacy and fill it, as they do for any other serious health issue. And they can travel for business and go on vacation.

As many of you know, as I write this, there is an epidemic within a pandemic going on in this country. More than 100,000 people died of an overdose last year. Even people who had been using heroin for years have begun to die, because it is now being mixed with fentanyl. Someone I know was very anxious and upset and asked a friend for a pill. Supposedly, it was Xanax. But it was a street version of Xanax mixed with fentanyl. He died.

Fortunately—what a word to use—because many of the people dying are white, what is happening is seen as a health crisis and not a criminal justice issue. Naloxone is now widely available and free in many areas. If you work with clients who might take a fentanyl-laced pill by accident, you may want to advise them to have naloxone on hand.

Chantix (varenicline) and Zyban (bupropion) have both been shown to be helpful to people trying to quit smoking. Even though smoking continues to be the leading preventable cause of death in the United States, both drugs are rarely advertised on television.

More recently, tirzepatide (Mounjaro) and semaglutide (Ozempic) have come on the market to help people lose weight. For some obesity patients, no amount of CBT or lifestyle changes has any impact. In those cases, medication can have a significant effect. Given that obesity is a health risk and inexpensive food is available in many countries, this medication may be a lifesaver for some patients.

Should Your Client Try PAT, KAT, MDMA, Ayahuasca, Psilocybin Mushrooms, or . . . ?

Again, what does your client want to do and why? Psychedelic-assisted therapy (PAT), ketamine-assisted therapy (KAT), and MDMA (ecstasy; methylenedioxymethamphetamine) are now being used in treatment. In some parts of the United States this is becoming a very popular way to deal with depression and for people suffering from trauma. These chemicals offer hope, something that we know is crucial for change and moving on in life.

It may help to ask your client: What is your goal? What are you hoping will happen? Who will be with you or who will be your "guide"? Where and when are you going to try it? The research results are mixed. As with other chemicals, it is impossible to know how one person will respond just because a group of participants in a research study did better than those who were given a placebo. It is, in fact, very difficult to do such a study and not come up with questionable results. Everyone who is given LSD or psilocybin knows that they have been given it and not a sugar pill. One study (Bogenschutz et al., 2022) compared the effect of psilocybin with the effect of an "active placebo." The researchers reported that those given psilocybin had significantly fewer heavy drinking days than those given diphenhydramine (Benadryl). But surely everyone given psilocybin knew they were given it and not an antihistamine. It is impossible to know what caused the reduction in heavy drinking days, knowing that they were in a research study and had been given an unusual chemical with unusual effects or the chemical itself.

20 Nonmedical Alternatives

Fortunately, we now know that there are many ways to affect our neurochemistry and the way our brain is functioning besides taking medications or something like MDMA or mushrooms. Below is a list of alternative ways that your client can use to affect their neurochemistry. Given the society that they are in, they may very strongly prefer to take a pill. It is much easier than almost anything else, and some pills alter the way people feel almost immediately, which is untrue of every alternative on this list. But almost none of the alternatives have unpleasant side effects, very few people get addicted to any of them, and they are all easy to stop, in most case without withdrawal. On the other hand, none of them alone will help someone sufficiently who is truly in need of medication.

People who are miserable are usually unmotivated. You want to be careful how you suggest something that might in fact be very helpful but may sound useless. That could injure your working alliance. As noted in chapters 7 and 8, restarting something that has helped in the past may be the best place to begin. Medications may help increase their motivation to do so. Consequently, a combination may be what is needed.

1. **Religious Rituals:** Praying, including repetitive prayers, such as saying Hail Marys and using a rosary, fasting, making offerings, pilgrimages, and other rituals, such as lighting a candle, all affect how people feel, think, and behave. That is probably one reason that such rituals have been embraced by so many people over so many years. They produce neurochemical changes.

2. **Dancing:** Throughout the world and historically for thousands of years, dance— American Indian dances, whirling dervishes, Sri Lankan Kandyan dances, and so on— have played a key role in almost all communities. More recently it is beginning to be studied by researchers (e.g., McCrary et al., 2021).

3. **Baking:** Some readers may think that I'm joking, but baking (and cooking) causes clients to think ahead, into the future, about something that will be enjoyable, that is, eating whatever they're making. Such thinking lifts people's spirits, that is, it causes beneficial neurochemical changes and probably physiological changes, as well. Baking also involves body movement, which is also very helpful in that it creates other neurochemical changes and affects metabolism, heart rate, and so forth. If your clients wind up sharing what they have made with others, that is a plus, too.

4. **Caffeine:** Some of your clients may be in your office because they consume too much caffeine. Caffeine may contribute to or even cause their generalized anxiety, social anxiety, and panic attacks. However, many people benefit from a little caffeine throughout the day. According to the federal government, 400 mg are okay. But that guideline ignores important individual differences, for example, how much your client weighs and how quickly or slowly they metabolize caffeine. For clients who are suffering from anxiety, even 200 mg may cause problems; 400 mg definitely will. Some people can't tolerate caffeine at all. Others get moderate amounts from sodas, green tea, eating chocolate, or taking a caffeine pill.

   In some ways, caffeine is not much different from psychotropic medications. It is just not as powerful and, when taken in moderation, has no effect on sexual performance or other negative side effects. In many people, it has a half-life of four hours. That means that half of it is gone in four hours and three-quarters in eight hours. A client who drinks a large Starbucks in the morning and then nothing else the rest of day and then complains of being tired is not taking into account that most of the caffeine has left their system by late afternoon. For them, it makes more sense to consume small amounts several times throughout the day. The amount of caffeine in popular drinks varies considerably (see Table 19.1).

5. **Chewing Gum:** It should not come as a surprise that chewing gum affects our neurochemistry (Kamiya et al., 2010). Otherwise, millions of people would not chew gum. Masticating may be one of the sources of pleasure in eating. Chewing improves reaction times, attention, and memory without taking a pill.

Table 19.1.

Drink	Caffeine level (mg)
Starbucks, 12 oz.	260
A standard cup of coffee	95 to 130
Red Bull, 8 oz.	80
Black tea, 8 oz.	47
Coke, 12 oz.	34
Green tea, 8 oz.	28

6. **Daydreaming:** Daydreaming, also referred to as self-generated thought in the research literature, has been found to involve many different regions of the brain (Fox et al., 2016). For many people, daydreaming and fantasizing help them cope throughout the day. Unfortunately, some people develop "maladaptive daydreaming," that is, daydreaming taken to an extreme where it is no longer helpful or adaptive. Initially, it may have helped them cope with anxiety, depression, and trauma. But then it impedes emotional, personal, academic, and professional growth and injures relationships. Consequently, it may be wise to ask your client whether daydreaming has been a problem. If so, encouraging daydreaming may not be advised.

7. **Exercise:** Exercise speeds up the heart, changes neurochemistry, and may, in the long run, be very beneficial for the entire body (Basso et al., 2022). I joke—but it not really a joke—that it is the cheapest form of antidepression, antianxiety "medication" available.

8. **Light:** Many people use light boxes to help them manage seasonal affective disorder (SAD), including anxiety, low mood, insomnia, hypersomnia, and social withdrawal (Choukroun & Geoffroy, 2019). In Finland, some university health centers provide light lamps for students to use for 30 to 60 minutes each morning.

9. **Meditation:** As I discussed in chapter 8, there are many forms of meditation. Some are specifically designed to calm down the brain. Loving-kindness meditation is designed to help people become more compassionate toward themselves and others. Some forms, perhaps all, affect neurochemistry (Mosini et al., 2019).

10. **Nicotine:** It is strange that nicotine is seen as benign. Perhaps marketing is behind that myth. According to one large study (Mishra et al., 2015), "Nicotine is well known to have serious systemic side effects in addition to being highly addictive. It adversely affects the heart, reproductive system, lung, kidney etc. Many studies have consistently demonstrated its carcinogenic potential" (p. 25). Most people continue to believe that it is the chemicals in the smoke of cigarettes that are the major cause of cancer. That may be the *major* cause. But nicotine is carcinogenic. Using a patch or vaping probably lowers the risk, but it does not eliminate it. Also, as is well known, nicotine is very addictive. Consequently, it is not a good method of changing one's neurochemistry.

11. **Reality Shifting:** "Reality shifting" (RS) has become popular on the internet (Somer et al., 2021). It is based on thousands of years of study in India and elsewhere into how to use the mind to create "entities," which, depending on whether you are a believer or a skeptic, is either seen as a hallucination or an actual alter being. Either way, RS probably also alters neurochemistry, although there is no research looking into this question to date. Whether it may entail risk is also unknown.

12. **Self-Help Meetings:** Many people report that going to self-help meetings—SMART Recovery, AA, Recovery Dharma—makes them feel better. If they feel better, their neurochemistry has changed.

13. **Sleep Hygiene:** People are finally beginning to realize that if they don't give up other activities to give their body enough time to sleep and rest, they will eventually become ill, physically, psychologically, or both. Wearables can help to monitor how much sleep they are getting—or not getting.

14. **Healthier Eating:** "Garbage in, garbage out" is a well-known saying in the computer world. If you put poor software or data in, you shouldn't expect good results out. The same is true for eating. Unfortunately, unhealthy foods are also inexpensive foods, and many people in the United States do not have access to healthy food.

15. **Sunlight:** Not surprisingly, many people find that they feel better after taking a walk outside, especially when it is a sunny day. Exposure to sunlight affects mood and cognitive

functioning (Kent et al., 2009). Ninety-five percent of serotonin is outside the brain and found in many parts of the body.

16. **Transcranial Magnetic Stimulation (TMS) and Electroconvulsive Therapy (ECT):** Many years ago, the "chemical imbalance" theory took off with the help of pharmaceutical companies, and research into how to affect neuroelectricity in the brain almost disappeared. That is still the case today, but some people are finding TMS helpful and ECT continues to be used.

    TMS and accelerated TMS have been both shown to be effective with depression, GAD, and PTSD (e.g., Cirillo et al., 2019; Sonmez et al., 2019). TMS does not require anesthesia and, unlike ECT, is not designed to produce seizures, although very rarely unintended seizures have been reported.

    No one really knows how ECT works. It is used on approximately 100,000 people per year. One recent review concluded: "There is no evidence that ECT is effective for . . . severely depressed people, or for suicidal people, people who have unsuccessfully tried other treatments first, involuntary patients, or adolescents. Given the high risk of permanent memory loss and the small mortality risk, this longstanding failure to determine whether or not ECT works means that its use should be immediately suspended" (Read et al., 2020, p. 1). But this conclusion is based on group data and has been strongly criticized by other researchers (Cattaneo et al., 2022; Meechan et al., 2022). As a result, at this point in time, it is for your client to decide. They may correctly believe from past ECTs with good outcomes that it works for them, or they may want to try ECT because everything else has failed.

17. **Travel:** People who love to travel say that one-third of the fun is thinking about the trip before actually leaving. Thinking about pleasant things like visiting a foreign country, having sex, going out to eat, and so on all produce dopamine, and a bit more dopamine makes us feel a bit better.

18. **VACI:** Many years ago, Albert Ellis urged people to develop a vital absorbing interest. SMART Recovery participants added a C to make it vital absorbing creative interest (VACI). It's not easy to start a VACI for people who are depressed or have been addicted to porn, video gaming, or a chemical. Initially, they cannot get enthused or motivated about almost anything else. But it is critically important that they begin to develop activities that are ongoing and reasonably enjoyable. Encouraging clients to try to reconnect with their innate curiosity may help get their dopamine system going again. Help them make a list of possible activities that they could explore, such as baking, music making, working with children or consulting on a start-up. Without absorbing interests, no medication is probably going to work over the long run.

19. **Movement:** "Movement is the best medicine," according to one doctor, even though, obviously, for some situations, it is not the "best." Movement lubricates joints, increases metabolism, improves balance. Pilates, tai chi, and taekwondo are only three of many movement arts that can effectively compliment cognitive, emotive, and interpersonal approaches.

20. **Music:** Historically, people in many parts of the world have used music to help them spiritually and psychologically. Tabla music in India and blues music in the United States are just two examples (Koshimori & Thaut, 2019; de Witte et al., 2022).

Combined Therapy

Most readers probably combine many of the above to help keep their neurochemistry and their mood and cognitive functioning more stable. This may not be true for your clients. They may think that none of the above will have any real effect, so they do very few, if any, of the activities listed. They don't get much exercise, don't pay attention to how much sleep they get, don't eat in a healthy manner, don't have a VACI, don't practice any religious rituals, don't meditate, and so on. They watch TV and may do one or two of the above. For example, they may listen to music. But one activity is probably not sufficient, so then they look for what is widely advertised: alcohol, pot, and pharmaceutical drugs to soothe them.

Without realizing it, clients may be hoping that just coming to therapy and talking about their problems will do the trick. Unfortunately, that is probably not the case. But suggesting to a client that they need to do 10 things to live a reasonably stable life could be counterproductive. Instead of enhancing hope and motivation, the effect would be the opposite. The very idea of having to do so many things would probably be demoralizing. However, trying to add one activity between sessions, perhaps one that they have done in the past and that they have found helpful, would be effective.

There is no doubt that psychotherapy helps many people. But there are those who are not helped. In our effort to be more open to multicultural considerations, it is critically important that we be more open to combining our approaches with other approaches that our clients may have found helpful. Staying on track, not becoming depressed again or relapsing to some form of addictive behavior is never easy. And none of the activities are necessarily easy at the time (e.g., going to church, following doctor's orders, being part of a dance group, or baking banana bread). But together, with the support of other people—therapists, doctors, members of the group—many are able to make their lives more fulfilling and enjoyable. However, like the Buddha, who kept meditating for the 43 years that he continued to teach, everyone has to continue to work, to observe, to notice, to practice the skills that they have learned, and to sustain hope and the motivation to make a difference in their own lives and those of others.

Chapter 20

Build Your Practice, Protect Yourself, and Prevent Burnout

No doubt, counseling and therapy can be an extremely rewarding and enjoyable profession. They are creative—you must come up with a new combination of strategies for each individual client—and you're helping others. On the other hand, helping clients will often not be a simple matter, as many factors may be involved, some of which cannot be changed. Some clients may be "cured" in only a few sessions, perhaps even just one. But some clients will return again and again over the years. It is important for counselors to protect themselves from becoming disheartened, discouraged, and demoralized. If they honor that what they are trying to do is sometimes difficult but important, they will do better over time.

WHAT CAN YOU DO?

Build Your Practice

To have enough clients, you have to get known and you should have a specialty. The two best specialties may be anxiety disorders and depression, because everyone suffers from some level of anxiety, and people, in general, seem to be more anxious than they were a few decades ago. People who suffer from depression tend to have repeated bouts even if they are fairly spaced out, so you might wind up working with someone for a very long time. In addition, if you help clients with either their anxiety or their depression, low-grade or major, they will be very appreciative and sing your praises, and maybe even refer people to you. Sports psychology is also a growing specialty, and if you're athletic and like working with athletes, that might be a good choice for you.

I chose to specialize in addictions for a variety of reasons, one of them being that addictions lie on the cusp between automatized, conditioned behavior and reflective, intentional behavior. People can't seem to control their behavior in certain circumstances and that aggravates them. But they are often very ambivalent about changing. Usually, they like some aspect of the behavior, be it drinking a lot of alcohol or watching too much porn. They may be appreciative if you help them get on a much better track, but they may not.

You can't keep up on the research on everything, so it is better to focus on one or two specialties, perhaps related, at the most. Join your local, county, or state professional associations and perhaps your national one, and then join the divisions or significant interest groups of your specialty. Go to their meetings even if you are a bit introverted and hate such social gatherings. People have to get to know you. Most counselors and therapists work around dinner and lunch time, but it is still a good idea to have a meal or coffee with people, especially if you are new in the neighborhood.

I helped found SMART Recovery. I thought AA and other 12-step programs were great for the people who liked them, but when I looked at the research, I found that most people did not resonate with them, only about 5%–15%. That left a lot of people out there who were looking for help. SMART also appeals to about 5%–15% of the people who initially come to a meeting, so other kinds of groups are needed.

SMART helped me get known in my community. I was asked to give talks at hospitals and colleges. I never took as a private client someone I met in a SMART meeting, but sometimes someone in a meeting would refer a friend or family member. Working at the institute also got me many referrals.

A successful professional colleague who works in a smallish community put his office in a medical center. That way he got referrals from the doctors, chiropractors, and physical therapists who also worked there. He also noted that someone could park their car in front of the center, and no one would know they were going for counseling. They might as easily be going to some other professional. He also did not put a big sign out in front for the same reason. He gave free talks in high schools and middle schools and got referrals from their guidance departments.

As I noted at the very beginning of this book, when I was working with a depressed or suicidal client, I was surrounded by excellent clinicians with years of experience, which made me much more comfortable, especially in the first several years of my practice.

I have also always put together panel discussions for my state and national professional organizations. For example, many years ago I put together the first panel on the treatment of gambling addiction for the APA convention. Being the organizer and moderator of a panel discussion gives you a reason to contact some of the top people in the field. You yourself don't have to know very much, and it will motivate you to read material that you might ordinarily not read.

That first panel also helped me decide whether I wanted to specialize in treating gamblers. Not surprisingly, it turned out that they are often in awful financial shape and as a man with a family, I couldn't afford to give my services away. Of course, initially I took insurance, but then, gradually as I got more clients, I stopped taking insurance, even though I continued taking Medicare clients for many years. SMART Recovery encourages people with all kinds of addictions to attend, so this was my way of providing some free services for people who could not afford mine and didn't have insurance.

I advertise in *Psychology Today*, have a website (https://cbtplusglobal.com/), and am active on LinkedIn and some other social networks, but not a lot. If I were younger, I would be much more active. You may also want to consider hiring a practice-building consultant. It may be well worth it. You may be a very good counselor or psychotherapist but awful at marketing. If you recognize that that is the case and can't seem to increase the time you spend on marketing, then hiring a consultant makes sense.

Protect Yourself

The following are six key ways to help protect yourself as a clinician.

1. Always have a "supervisor," someone with experience whom you can consult. The word "supervisor" is appropriate in a training setting. Your supervisor is literally supervising

the way you are doing therapy with your clients. You meet weekly and discuss clients and particularly difficult issues.

Later, if you are in independent practice, it is important to continue to have someone you can call on when you find yourself working with a difficult client and may be confused as to what you should do next. When I worked at the institute, I went to talk to the executive director, Dr. Kristene Doyle. She is probably 30 years younger than I am, but is very experienced, smart, and direct. I've worked a long time, and I like to think that I'm a good clinician, but she often made suggestions that I should have thought of myself but hadn't. In addition, answering her questions helped me gain insight into problems that I was grappling with. She told me several times that she appreciated that she could always count on me to come to talk with her the minute I suspected that there might be a problem, rather than waiting until something serious developed. Young people at the institute didn't always do that. Maybe they were thinking (or telling themselves) something like:

I should know how to do this.

If I go speak to my supervisor, I may reveal how inexperienced I really am.

I don't want to look stupid in front of my supervisor.

I can handle this.

This will blow over.

But when it doesn't "blow over" and blows up instead, then what?

At the institute, the terms "transference" and "countertransference" are not used. However, talking to someone else sometimes helps clarify that a practitioner is feeling something that is getting in the way of treating a client effectively.

2. Before you talk to your supervisor, make sure you have paper and pen by your side or a laptop with you. Do not have such an important conversation riding home in a taxi at night. Sit down and take notes. Then put those notes in your file. That will help protect you if something does go wrong.

3. Do what you agreed to do with your supervisor. This is not the time to avoid or procrastinate. If you do see yourself avoiding, go talk again. A good supervisor has dealt with avoidance before. Avoidance is not so rare in our profession. We like to help people feel better. Sometimes what we need to do is refer the client out to some other professional. They, the clients, may feel as if they have been "fired." That won't make them feel better but doing the right thing—referring out—will make you feel better in the long run, especially if you avoid a professional train wreck.

4. Join a professional organization that has a lawyer available for consultation. Consult with them if you and your supervisor think that that would be a good idea. Again, take notes on that call. Put them in your file. And carefully do what the lawyer says you should do. Document that, too.

5. If appropriate, call your insurance company for advice, and document that call, as well.

6. When you come to renew your insurance, if you have even a slight sense that you might have a serious problem with a particular client in the future, call them and ask them how to answer the questions required for renewal. If you answer as if there is no potential problem on the horizon, they may later refuse to cover a claim because, according to them, you did not answer honestly.

Prevent Burnout

It is very sad if someone who is good in the field or could be good quits because of burnout. To prevent burnout:

1. Don't see too many clients. No doubt, one clinician will be able to see more clients than another and still function well. How many you can see and still listen carefully and ask good questions will no doubt depend on your individual capacities. Of course, some clinics and hospitals may require you see more people than you can reasonably work effectively with. Although just listening in an empathetic manner may help many people, it may make some people narcissistic because, in a sense, they are encouraged to go on and on talking about what has happened to them. As I've said before, that's unfortunate because such behavior outside a therapy room will injure relationships, and relationships are key to a client's overall psychological well-being.

2. As I suggested in chapter 3, take notes during the session. This is especially important if your workplace requires you to see a lot of clients. Many young counselors and therapists have been trained not to take notes during a session. Where did this idea come from? Freud took notes. The assumption, I think, is that if you are taking notes, you cannot listen in the same way. Listening and writing is difficult. And it is important to make sure you are not writing to avoid really listening or to avoid having to say something. On the other hand, if you take notes during the session, when the client leaves, you will be finished. If you don't write your notes during your session and wait for the session to end, what happens if your supervisor wants to see you or you have to meet some friends after work? Then having to write the notes will be hanging over your head all night. And what about the guilt? Surely you are not going to remember accurately after even a few hours pass. What other clients have said to you will interfere with that. Too much guilt and you will begin to hate your work. You'll burn out. How can that help your clients?

3. Occasionally, a client says something in a unique way. Writing notes during the sessions allows you to capture exactly what a client says in the moment. That may be very helpful a month or six months later. If you don't write it when your client says it, you probably won't get it exactly right.

4. Take a 20-minute power nap in the middle of your day. Half the people in the world love naps and half hate them. If you are in the latter group, 20 minutes of meditation may work just as well, but many people can get into the habit of a 20-minute nap. You won't feel as if you have been asleep, but 20 minutes will eliminate the chemical in your brain, adenosine, that makes you sleepy, and, later, you won't have to stop yourself from yawning in front of a client and you won't feel as exhausted when you get home.

5. Do not see too many people back to back.

Textbox 20.1. Research Note #10: Can You Work Well with Every Client?

Counselors and therapists should not assume that they can be helpful to everyone. That is one of several possible takeaways from a study done by Kraus and colleagues (2011). That research also suggests that some therapists are definitely better in one problem domain than others and no therapist is good in all. Their study included 6960 patients and 696 therapists. Using Kraus's Treatment Outcome Package (TOP), they assessed the effectiveness of treatment and of the therapists over 12 domains (e.g., work functioning, violence, social functioning, panic/anxiety, substance abuse, depression, sleep, and quality of life). Some therapists were "exponentially" better than others and some were much worse. They found that approximately a quarter of all of the therapists were good in five to six domains.

For example, 67% were effective with clients suffering from depression but only 43% for panic/anxiety. Nearly all therapists were effective in some areas, but none were effective in all. Unfortunately, some therapists, from 0.3 to 16% depending on the domain, were harmful to their clients. That is, the clients left treatment worse off than they began.

This study is also interesting because 52% of the clients were non-white (71% of the therapists were white) and from lower-income classes, that is, 51% reported income of 0–10 thousand dollars and 18% 10–20 thousand. Perhaps that might partly explain the "harmful" therapy in this study. Many people choose the therapist and the kind of therapy they engage in. That may have not been the case for all of the people in this study, and some people didn't find the form of therapy they were offered worked for them.

10 Typical Unhelpful Thoughts Counselors and Therapists May Have

Unfortunately, we clinicians can think unhelpful thoughts as well as our clients. Fortunately, we have tools to help us when we do. During workshops, I have collected unhelpful beliefs that clinicians find themselves thinking. The following are the most typical.

1. This person will never change.
2. This is pointless and a waste of my time.
3. I should be able to help this person.
4. My supervisor or my client's family members will think I'm not a good clinician.
5. I should have gone into a different profession.
6. I'm a failure.
7. It's hopeless. I'll never be a good counselor/therapist.
8. I don't know what to do, as I should.
9. I never do anything well.
10. No one cares.

How would you deal with such beliefs? Which do you hear most often? As I noted in chapter 14, writing a list of the most typical unhelpful ideas that your brain tosses up is a very effective first step. You can become familiar with them. Becoming familiar with them will lessen their power. They are not exactly old friends, but when they show up, you will recognize them. You won't be caught completely by surprise. More importantly, you can learn how to deal with them effectively. In the beginning, you may be quite flummoxed when your brain suggests, *F*ck it. This is pointless.* Learning the best way to deal with such thoughts/feelings results in your being prepared.

If your brain is tossing up something like *I should be able to help this person*, what could you think that might help you?

Maybe: *It would be great if I could help everybody, but I can't. Nobody can help everybody* or *There is no law of the universe that says I (or any other therapist) should be able to help everybody. What can I do that has helped in the past?*

RAIN (see chapter 11) may be helpful, as well. Talking to your supervisor may be very important, too. Figuring out what helps you take care of yourself is key to working well. What combination of tools, strategies, etc., will help you? Getting some sleep, getting together with friends, a walk in the woods, a bike ride, baking, dancing, making or listening to music, eating some chocolate, making yourself a cup of tea . . . what will help you work successfully and enjoy your work most of the time?

Individual versus Group

Although some clients won't feel comfortable sharing in a group and, for that reason, will opt for individual therapy, no evidence exists that individual therapy is superior to group therapy. Moreover, group therapy is almost always less expensive than individual therapy. Janis and her colleagues (2021) reviewed 42 studies between 1990 and 2018 of group therapy for depression and for bipolar disorder and found that group therapy for depression was superior to the treatment as usual (TAU) and the waitlist conditions. It was also as effective as medication. Dropout rates did not differ.

In a study of group versus individual CPT for PTSD in active-duty military personnel, Resick and her associates (2017) found "no differences in remission or severity of PTSD at the 6-month follow-up. Symptoms of depression and suicidal ideation did not differ significantly between formats" (p. 28). Note, however, that 50% of the participants still had PTSD at the end of the study, perhaps because the intervention was too short (i.e., two times per week for six weeks).

In another study (Murphy et al., 2020), 42 perpetuators of intimate partner violence who sought treatment at a community domestic violence agency were randomly assigned to either CBT integrated with MI (ICBT) or group CBT (GBCT). The men and their partners went for 20 sessions of ICBT or 20 weeks of GCBT. They evaluated their relationship every three months for a year. Attendance was significantly higher in ICBT, but the effectiveness of GCBT was equal or better than ICBT. The authors note that the group setting may have been more effective because "the group may facilitate greater subsequent engagement through role modeling and positive social influence. Ambivalence may be more readily resolved through observation of group members experiencing benefits from their change efforts rather than through protracted MI with an individual therapist" (p. 2862).

Long-Term versus Short-Term Therapy

Insufficient research evidence exists to determine which is better, short- or long-term therapy. Moreover, if such evidence did exist, would it be relevant for the individual sitting in your room? Such studies and results would be based on averages of group data. Individual differences would be lost. If your client wants to be in therapy for a long time, that should be their decision. Frank Gehry, the architect who has given us multiple beautiful buildings, such as the Guggenheim Museum in Bilboa and the IAC building on the West Side of Manhattan at 18th Street, reportedly has seen a therapist for more than 30 years. Perhaps it has helped him create such wonderful buildings for us to enjoy.

However, practitioners need to be mindful. Is the fact that they will make more money if clients come for more sessions influencing how they work with clients? In the past and even today, when a client suggests that they are thinking about stopping therapy, the clinician may suggest that the client is thinking about leaving therapy because they are "resistant." It would be too uncomfortable for them to move forward and uncover more painful material. In some cases, that might be the case. But it might also be true that the therapy is not working or that it has already been helpful, and the client is correct to stop, perhaps for a while.

I have seen some clients for more than 20 years. Most of those clients are managing a genuine bipolar disorder. I see some on a more or less regular basis, once per month, to help them maintain, as much as possible, stability in their lives. I see others intermittently, usually only when a crisis arises. A combined, integrated approach has helped them stay out of hospitals for the most part and in some cases have jobs and even get married. I see a client, Frida, about once per month. I have seen her for more than 20 years. In addition to seeing me, she sees a psychiatrist, takes her medication regularly, swims three times a week, goes to church and prays daily, has a dog and walks it, organizes and takes trips, and calls me when something bad has happened or she is having a particularly difficult time with her husband, who is a good, kind man but has difficulties himself.

Telehealth

The pandemic brought loss, pain, and tragedy to many people, but it also finally made telehealth acceptable and available to everyone. In addition, the research results are clear. Telehealth works as effectively as face-to-face therapy (Greenwood et al., 2022; Krzyzaniak et al., 2021; Nauphal et al., 2021; Scott et al., 2022). It also makes counseling and therapy available to many more people than before. Researchers and clinicians are also learning how to use computer technology to interact with their clients in ways that go beyond just seeing each other and talking. For example, in one study (Stewart et al., 2020), the telehealth outreach program (TOP) in South Carolina, games were created that could be played interactively using the screen-sharing function of the video program. TOP provided services to 70 young people in underserved communities. Thirty-four percent of the children and 57% of the caregivers requested that the services be delivered in Spanish. Of the 88.6% of the children who completed the program, 97% no longer met the diagnostic criteria for PTSD.

What We Gained from the Pandemic

People who may be parents with children or have two jobs are finally able to access help. Currently, I run two free online meetings. On average 15 to 20 people participate via audio or both audio and video, but 60–100 people attend from all over the globe, including Chicago, Berlin, London, and Cairo. Many have their cameras turned off. This may be because stigma regarding addictions is still widespread and intense or because they're at work. I like to think that they may be benefiting. They can see that it is quite common for people to grapple with difficult emotional, behavioral, and thinking problems. One-half of the meeting is spent checking in and sharing. During the other half, we do some kind of skills-based exercise. The exercises demonstrate other ways to manage life's problems without addictive behaviors.

What We Have Lost

I can't walk out, meet my client, go up in the elevator, and make "small talk," all of the time observing and assessing. But I think I've become quite good at doing the same thing during the first few minutes of a virtual appointment, carefully paying attention to any subtle differences in tone and nonverbal body language.

What We Did Not Gain

I work in New York, one mile from New Jersey, where some of my clients live. Is it legal for me to do telehealth with them while they are sitting in New Jersey, and I'm sitting in New York? I called my insurance company. I was told, "As long as you comply with all of the laws of the State of New York, you are covered." Unfortunately, the laws of New York are not clear.

In contrast, the New Jersey Psychological Association is very clear. I cannot do so. But during the pandemic, a special law was passed in New Jersey, and I was able to request a special license, under COVID, to work with people in that state, and I did. But that law has expired. Something similar is true for social workers and mental health counselors. The pandemic did not change that. You will have to decide, perhaps after consulting coworkers in your state, your supervisor, and your insurance company whether you are comfortable working with people outside your state.

Can you legally provide services to someone overseas? The insurance company gave me the same answer, but there is no way of knowing. Besides insurance coverage considerations, if you were to talk to someone in India, and they become suicidal and needed to be hospitalized, do you know who to contact? In some cases, you may know a psychiatrist in a foreign city, and you are comfortable providing services to people in that city. But it is very likely that such a client would be wealthy. They might also have money in New York City banks and lawyers here, as well. Do you want to take the risk if you are not sure your insurance policy covers you that something may happen, and you get sued? At the very least, it seems wise never to work with someone virtually without having emergency contact information for someone in their life and, preferably, the number of a psychiatrist or internist where they live.

Sometimes I talk to clients outside of New York State on the basis of the ethical concept of "continuation of care." It is not ethical for me to refuse to talk to a client of mine who is requesting a session. That is, it is not ethical for me to refuse to continue to "see" the person just because they are not, at the time, in New York State. But I cannot use that reason for weeks on end. The client has to find someone local to continue therapy. That is unfortunate. Perhaps some of the readers of this book will become involved in the movement to change those guild-based laws.

Give Back to Help a More Diverse Group of People

Once you have a license from your state, you have a license to make money. You probably won't make as much as your plumber or doctor, but, if you're willing to work hard, you have an assured source of income for the rest of your life. If you have a state license, an insurance company or Medicare will reimburse your clients or pay you directly.

However, many potential clients don't have insurance and/or can't afford your fee. Many professionals in the field want to extend counseling services to underserved communities. To do so, as licensed therapists and counselors, we have to find ways to make our services available to such people. Some readers may have to work in jobs that require them to see more clients than is humanly possible and still do a good job, have a life outside of work, and perhaps raise a family. If that is your situation, you are probably already doing your part. But to expand our services to a more diverse clientele, consider devoting a percentage of your time and energy in the following ways.

1. Become a Medicaid provider. You won't get paid as well, but there are thousands of people on Medicaid who could benefit from your services.
2. Become a Medicare provider. Again, you may be paid less than you are paid by your other clients, but there is a great need. For many years, approximately 30% of my total client load were Medicare clients.
3. Provide low-fee counseling at a church, temple, or mosque or at a college in your community.

4. Work with a nonprofit such as SMART Recovery, AA, or NAMI, the National Alliance on Mental Illness. Learn to facilitate a free SMART Recovery online meeting (https://www.smartrecovery.org/). Training is very inexpensive and can be done online. In addition, you will probably learn something from every meeting you run, so this is not solely altruistic behavior.

Is Termination Appropriate?

What other profession "terminates" clients? Where did the word come from? Psychoanalysis was designed to help the unconscious become conscious and to restructure the personality of a client. It took a long time, many sessions per week, and when it was over, it is understandable that considerable attention would be paid to ending such a long, important relationship.

But most modern therapists and counselors are not trying to restructure their client's personality. They are focused on helping clients change the way they feel, think, and behave during difficult times in their lives.

As I mentioned before, I've seen some clients on and off for 20 or 30 years, but I have seen some clients for only two or three sessions. Many people with bipolar disorder, PDD, MDD, and some with addictions do not get over their problems. They learn how to manage them. But sometimes life throws them so many curveballs at once that they need help to stay on track or get back on track. They know that they can always call me. That is the case for the other professionals in their life (i.e., their internist, dentist, lawyer, and cleaning person). Again, why do counselors and therapists end—"terminate"—their relationships with clients? It does not make sense.

Of course, if I have not seen someone for seven years and can hardly remember who they are, I shred the file. But there are files that I have kept for years. In one case, a 75-year-old woman appeared. I had seen her 23 years before when she was having difficulties in her marriage. She said, "You cured me then [her words, said with a big smile], and I hope you can cure me now." Her husband of 50 years had passed away and after two years and against the advice of her friends, she had fallen for a known womanizer.

"What was wrong with Alice [not her real name]?" she asked, referring to herself in the third person. "How could she have been so stupid? And now I am acting like a 17-year-old all over again. I can't believe it. I can't even walk down the street where he usually parks his car. I hate going to my community center. I might see him!"

She had temporarily lost her bearings. We worked together for only four sessions. She was not the first older person I had seen who had fallen in love, had gotten cheated on, and was devastated by it. I told her about those people, without, of course, mentioning anything specific. We talked about how she had generally run her life in an intelligent manner, but she also had made some mistakes, like this one. Could she accept that? She eventually could. She even could begin to laugh at herself, clearly a good sign. I was glad I had never "terminated" her.

In another case, 20 years after I had helped someone with marital issues, he reappeared in my office. At age 60, he was tired of always being anxious and always second-guessing his decisions. He had managed to have a good career as an internist and had raised two children who had both graduated from college and were on their feet. His wife had been reading *The Body Keeps the Score*, and she told him she thought he was suffering from a traumatic upbringing, although neither she nor he had brought that up in their previous sessions. I found my old notes. His father had died when he was 12, and his mother had always been critical and drank a lot when he was young, and still did. We began to work together again.

Textbox 20.2. Case—Maya: Remembering the Positive

Maya, a young, attractive woman, came into the office complaining of depression and anxiety. At 40, she had broken up with her second, serious partner and was wondering if she would ever find someone she could be with in a long-term relationship. She came from Southeast Asia and regularly sent money home to support her mother and, according to her, her "pain in the ass" brother who not only had never worked but also threatened her on her last trip home.

She was a successful researcher working in a medical lab, but clearly undervalued herself and her ability to be successful. This was so although she was the first and only person in her family to graduate from college, let alone get a PhD. She consistently won grants for the lab where she worked and had published several articles in well-respected journals.

I was struck by the discrepancy between what she had managed to do with her life, especially given the poor neighborhood that she grew up in and her family problems, and how she felt about herself. But I was not surprised. That is very common. Those who believe in the neurochemical or medical model see this as proof that there is a lack of some neurotransmitter, perhaps serotonin or dopamine, that causes people to feel so down despite everything being relatively good in their life. And maybe that is correct, but perhaps that "imbalance" can be corrected without medicine, so I asked, "How would you feel about writing a list of good things that you have done or achieved in your life? Sometimes it can help if people focus on the positive in therapy not always on what is going wrong."

Not surprisingly, she looked puzzled, but her face and body language suggested that she liked something about the idea.

"Okay. I'll try," she said.

When she came in the next week, and I asked her about it, she smiled, and said, "You know, I was so sure I couldn't do it, that when I got to my car, I sat there and started my list. Actually, I came up with 10 things right there. I was so surprised."

I could see how happy she was.

That session we started talking about her relationships and why she thought they had all been problematic. The second I said "problematic" I saw her face change, and I saw her eyeballs move to the right.

"What just flashed through your mind?" I asked.

"What do you mean?" she answered.

"Well, often when we talk about something that is upsetting to us, we have glimpses, tiny videoclips, of something that happened in our childhood. When I was 10, at an important moment in a baseball game, I struck out. I was not a very good player, and that just drove that fact home, to use a baseball analogy. Sometimes, when I get stuck or things are going badly, that scene, me walking back from home plate, feeling crushed, flashes through my mind. What flashed through yours?"

She looked uncomfortable. I sat and held my pen still and looked away for a moment.

"My father abused me when I was thirteen," she said. Nothing more.

"Oh, I'm very sorry to hear that. You can tell me a bit more if you want to, but you don't have to if you don't want to. That's up to you."

I sat quietly, alternatively looking at her and then away, to give her some space and time to think.

"No. It's okay. I guess I better talk about it." And she did. The abuse lasted from age 13 to 16. Her mother and father were separated, and it happened when she visited her father. She didn't think her mother ever knew. She didn't visit him often.

I did not ask any questions then about what specifically had happened. I let her share what she wanted to at that time.

Again, I don't think any manual or book can tell you the exact best way to proceed, although learning about cognitive processing therapy and other forms of therapy for trauma may help. Clearly, how you look and sit has an impact. Avoiding talking about it may increase the feelings of shame about what happened: "Even my therapist doesn't want to hear about it." But spending more time on something like that than a client wants can also be a major mistake. Clients need to feel that they have control over that kind of conversation.

After she talked for a while, I asked her, "How do you feel about all this now?"

"I don't know. I don't think about it much."

"Well, if we want to better understand what is going on in your relationships, we should probably talk more about this, but that is always up to you, how much and when you talk about it in session."

"Okay," she said, and we started to talk about something else, but we returned to her abuse many times, sometimes only very briefly. She seemed always to get involved with women who were less professionally successful and more emotionally troubled. How did she think what happened in her adolescence might be contributing to that? She had no idea, so I suggested, just as a hypothesis, that she felt helpless and powerless when she was a teenager in the face of a more powerful person, so it was important to always date someone less successful and less powerful psychologically. She thought that was possible.

At about that point, I asked her why she didn't have a better, more highly paid position. She didn't understand my question. I knew that people in her field were often paid $80K. She was only making $40K. I suggested that she didn't feel that good about herself—powerless, helpless—so she didn't dare apply for a better job. I told her about a specific job that I knew about. Not all stories in therapy end happily, but in her case, within a few months she applied, went for interviews, and got the job, at twice what she had been making!

At that point, she was not dating anyone, and we agreed that she would stop therapy for a while to focus on doing well at her new job and call me when she started dating someone again. Sometimes I ask, and I did then, "What do you think helped most in therapy?"

She smiled and asked, "Do you remember the very first assignment you gave me, the one I thought I couldn't do? That really startled me. I somehow just thought we would talk about the negative in therapy."

References

Adler, A. (2002). *The collected clinical works of Alfred Adler* (Vol. 1). Alfred Adler Institute.

Aibar-Almazán, A., Hita-Contreras, F., Cruz-Díaz, D., de la Torre-Cruz, M., Jiménez-García, J. D., & Martínez-Amat, A. (2019). Effects of Pilates training on sleep quality, anxiety, depression and fatigue in postmenopausal women: A randomized controlled trial. *Maturitas, 124*, 62–67.

Angell, M. (2011a). The epidemic of mental illness: Why? *New York Review of Books, 58*(11), 20–22.

Angell, M. (2011b). The illusions of psychiatry. *New York Review of Books, 58*(12), 20–22.

Arntz, A. (2012). Imagery rescripting as a therapeutic technique: Review of clinical trials, basic studies, and research agenda. *Journal of Experimental Psychopathology, 3*(2), 189–208.

Arora, S., Gonzalez, K. A., Abreu, R. L., & Gloster, C. (2022). Therapy can be restorative, but can also be really harmful: Therapy experiences of QTBIPOC clients. Psychotherapy, 59(4), 498–510. https://doi.org/10.1037/pst0000443

Barnett, J. E. (2011). Psychotherapist self-disclosure: Ethical and clinical considerations. *Psychotherapy, 48*(4), 315.

Basso, J. C., Oberlin, D. J., Satyal, M. K., O'Brien, C. E., Crosta, C., Psaras, Z., Metpally1\, A., & Suzuki, W. A. (2022). Examining the effect of increased aerobic exercise in moderately fit adults on psychological state and cognitive function. *Frontiers in Human Neuroscience, 16*, 375. https://doi.org/10.3389/fnhum.2022.833149

Bateson, G. (2000). Why do Frenchmen? In B. A. U. Levinson (Ed.), *Schooling the symbolic animal: Social and cultural dimensions of education* (pp. 62–65). Rowman & Littlefield.

Beck, A. T. (1975). *Cognitive therapy and the emotional disorders*. Meridian.

Bercik, P., Denou, E., Collins, J., Jackson, W., Lu, J., Jury, J., Deng, Y., Blennerhassett, P., Macri, J., McCoy, K. D., Verdu, E. F., & Collins, S. M. (2011). The intestinal microbiota affect central levels of brain-derived neurotropic factor and behavior in mice. *Gastroenterology, 141*(2), 599–609. https://doi.org/10.1053/j.gastro.2011.04.052

Berkowitz, S. J., Stover, C. S., & Marans, S. R. (2011). The child and family traumatic stress intervention: Secondary prevention for youth at risk of developing PTSD. *Journal of Child Psychology and Psychiatry, 52*(6), 676–85.

Bhikku, T. (2014). There is no self. *Tricycle, The Buddhist Review*. https://tricycle.org/magazine/there-no-self/

Bishop, F. M. (2018). Self-guided change: The most common form of long-term, maintained health behavior change. *Health Psychology Open, 5*(1), 2055102917751576. https://doi.org/10.1177/2055102917751576

Bogenschutz, M. P., Ross, S., Bhatt, S., Baron, T., Forcehimes, A. A., Laska, E., Mennenga, S. E., O'Donnell, K., Owens, L. T., Podrebarac, S., Rotrosen, J., Tonigan, J. S., & Worth, L. (2022). Percentage of heavy drinking days following psilocybin-assisted psychotherapy vs placebo in the treatment of adult patients with alcohol use disorder: A randomized clinical trial. *JAMA Psychiatry, 79*(10), 953–962. https://doi.org/10.1001/jamapsychiatry.2022.2096

Boren, J. J., Leventhal, A. M., & Pigott, H. E. (2009). Just how effective are antidepressant medications? Results of a major new study. *Journal of Contemporary Psychotherapy, 39,* 93–100.

Bowlby, J. (1979). The Bowlby-Ainsworth attachment theory. *Behavioral and Brain Sciences, 2*(4), 637–638.

Bradshaw, J. (1988). *Healing the shame that binds you.* Health Communications.

Bronson, P. (2013). *What should I do with my life?* Random House.

Brown, L. S. (2004). Feminist paradigms of trauma treatment. *Psychotherapy: Theory, Research, Practice, Training, 41*(4), 464–471. https://doi.org/10.1037/0033-3204.41.4.464

Buchanan, M. (2013). *Forecast: What physics, meteorology, and the natural sciences can teach us about economics.* Bloomsbury Publishing.

Bunton, R., Baldwin, S., Flynn, D., & Whitelaw, S. (2000). The "stages of change" model in health promotion: Science and ideology. *Critical Public Health, 10*(1), 55–70.

Burgess, D. J., Beach, M. C., & Saha, S. (2017). Mindfulness practice: A promising approach to reducing the effects of clinician implicit bias on patients. *Patient Education and Counseling, 100*(2), 372–376. https://doi.org/10.1016/j.pec.2016.09.005

Burns, D. D. (2000). *Feeling good* (2nd ed.). Harper.

Bynum, L., Griffin, T., Riding, D. L., Wynkoop, K. S., Anda, R. F., Edwards, V. J., . . . & Croft, J. B. (2010). Adverse childhood experiences reported by adults—five states, 2009. *Morbidity and Mortality Weekly Report, 59*(49), 1609–1613.

Calabria, B., Degenhardt, L., Briegleb, C., Vos, T., Hall, W., Lynskey, M., Callaghan, B., Rana, U., & McLaren, J. (2010). Systematic review of prospective studies investigating "remission" from amphetamine, cannabis, cocaine or opioid dependence. *Addictive Behaviors, 35*(8), 741–749.

Captari, L. E., Hook, J. N., Hoyt, W., Davis, D. E., McElroy-Heltzel, S. E., & Worthington, E. L. Jr. (2018). Integrating clients' religion and spirituality within psychotherapy: A comprehensive meta-analysis. *Journal of Clinical Psychology, 74*(11), 1938–1951.

Captari, L. E., Sandage, S. J., & Vandiver, R. A. (2022). Spiritually integrated psychotherapies in real-world clinical practice: Synthesizing the literature to identify best practices and future research directions. *Psychotherapy, 59*(3), 307–20. https://doi.org/10.1037/pst0000407

Carey, B., & Gebeloff, R. (2018, April 7). Many people taking antidepressants discover they cannot quit. *New York Times,* 7.

Carpenter, S. (2012). That gut feeling. *Monitor on Psychology, 43*(8), 50.

Castonguay, L. G., Eubanks, C. F., Goldfried, M. R., Muran, J. C., & Lutz, W. (2015). Research on psychotherapy integration: Building on the past, looking to the future. *Psychotherapy Research, 25*(3), 365–382.

Cattaneo, C. I., Ressico, F., Fornaro, M., Fazzari, G., & Perugi, G. (2022). The shocking attitude toward electroconvulsive therapy in Italy. *CNS Spectrums, 27*(2), 131–133.

Choukroun, J., & Geoffroy, P. A. (2019). Light therapy in mood disorders: A brief history with physiological insights. *Chronobiology in Medicine, 1*(1), 3–8.

Cirillo, P., Gold, A. K., Nardi, A. E., Ornelas, A. C., Nierenberg, A. A., Camprodon, J., & Kinrys, G. (2019). Transcranial magnetic stimulation in anxiety and trauma-related disorders: A systematic review and meta-analysis. *Brain and Behavior, 9*(6), e01284.

Clark, D. A., & Rhyno, S. (2005). Unwanted intrusive thoughts in nonclinical individuals: Implications for clinical disorders. In D. A. Clark (Ed.), *Intrusive thoughts in clinical disorders: Theory, research, and treatment* (pp. 1–29). Guilford Press.

Clear, J. (2018). *Atomic habits: An easy & proven way to build good habits & break bad ones.* Penguin.

Cody, G. W. (2018). The origins of integrative medicine—The first true integrators: Western States class of 1953. *Integrative Medicine: A Clinician's Journal, 17*(6), 12–16.

Conze, E. (1959). *Buddhism: Its essence and development.* Windhorse Publications.

Cooper, A. A., Kline, A. C., Graham, B., Bedard-Gilligan, M., Mello, P. G., Feeny, N. C., & Zoellner, L. A. (2017). Homework "dose," type, and helpfulness as predictors of clinical outcomes in prolonged exposure for PTSD. *Behavior Therapy, 48*(2), 182–194.

Cosci, F., & Chouinard, G. (2020). Acute and persistent withdrawal syndromes following discontinuation of psychotropic medications. *Psychotherapy and Psychosomatics, 89*(5), 283–306.

Cuijpers, P., Reijnders, M., & Huibers, M. J. (2019). The role of common factors in psychotherapy outcomes. *Annual Review of Clinical Psychology, 15*(1), 207–231.

Dalai Lama, Tutu, D., & Abrams, D. C. (2016). *The book of joy: Lasting happiness in a changing world.* Penguin.

Dalgleish, T., Black, M., Johnston, D., & Bevan, A. (2020). Transdiagnostic approaches to mental health problems: Current status and future directions. *Journal of Consulting and Clinical Psychology, 88*(3), 179–195. https://doi.org/10.1037/ccp0000482

David, D., Cristea, I., & Hofmann, S. G. (2018). Why cognitive behavioral therapy is the current gold standard of psychotherapy. *Frontiers in Psychiatry, 9.* https://doi.org/10.3389/fpsyt.2018.00004

Davis, D. E., DeBlaere, C., Brubaker, K., Owen, J., Jordan, T. A., Hook, J. N., & Van Tongeren, D. R. (2016). Microaggressions and perceptions of cultural humility in counseling. *Journal of Counseling & Development, 94*(4), 483–493.

Davis, M., Eshelman, E. R., & McKay, M. (2008). *The relaxation and stress reduction workbook.* New Harbinger Publications.

DeBlaere, C., Zelaya, D. G., Dean, J.-A. B., Chadwick, C. N., Davis, D. E., Hook, J. N., & Owen, J. (2023). Multiple microaggressions and therapy outcomes: The indirect effects of cultural humility and working alliance with Black, Indigenous, women of color clients. *Professional Psychology: Research and Practice, 54*(2), 115–124. https://doi.org/10.1037/pro0000497

de Botton, A. (2012). *How to think more about sex.* MacMillan.

Decker, S. E., Kiluk, B. D., Frankforter, T., Babuscio, T., Nich, C., & Carroll, K. M. (2016). Just showing up is not enough: Homework adherence and outcome in cognitive-behavioral therapy for cocaine dependence. *Journal of Consulting and Clinical Psychology, 84*(10), 907.

De Haan, K. L. B., Lee, C. W., Fassbinder, E., Van Es, S. M., Menninga, S., Meewisse, M. L., Rijkeboer, M., Kousemaker, M., & Arntz, A. (2020). Imagery rescripting and eye movement desensitisation and reprocessing as treatment for adults with post-traumatic stress disorder from childhood trauma: Randomised clinical trial. *British Journal of Psychiatry, 217*(5), 609–615.

DeRubeis, R. J., Siegle, G. J., & Hollon, S. D. (2008). Cognitive therapy versus medication for depression: Treatment outcomes and neural mechanisms. *Nature Reviews Neuroscience, 9*(10), 788–796.

de Witte, M., Pinho, A. D. S., Stams, G. J., Moonen, X., Bos, A. E., & van Hooren, S. (2022). Music therapy for stress reduction: A systematic review and meta-analysis. *Health Psychology Review, 16*(1), 134–159.

Dobson, K. S. (2021). A commentary on the science and practice of homework in cognitive behavioral therapy. *Cognitive Therapy and Research, 45*, 303–309.

Doidge, N. (2007). *The brain that changes itself: Stories of personal triumph from the frontiers of brain science.* Penguin.

dos-Santos-Silva, I., Gupta, S., Orem, J., & Shulman, L. N. (2022). Global disparities in access to cancer care. *Communications Medicine, 2*(1), 1–4.

Dryden, W. (1998). Understanding persons in the context of their problems: A rational emotive behaviour therapy perspective. In M. Bruch & F. W. Bond (Eds.), *Beyond diagnosis: Case formulation approaches in CBT* (pp. 43–64). Wiley.

Dweck, C. (2015). Carol Dweck revisits the growth mindset. *Education Week, 35*(5), 20–24.

Dweck, C. S. (1986). Motivational processes affecting learning. *American Psychologist, 41*(10), 1040.

Ehrenreich, B. (2009). *Bright-sided: How positive thinking is undermining America.* Metropolitan Books.

Ellis, A. (1962). *Reason and emotion in psychotherapy.* Lyle Stuart.

Ellis, A. (2019). *How to stubbornly refuse to make yourself miserable: About anything—yes, anything!* Hachette UK.

Ellis, A. (2003). Cognitive restructuring of the disputing of irrational beliefs. In W. T. O'Donohue & J. E. Fisher (Eds.), *Cognitive behavior therapy: Applying empirically supported techniques in your practice* (pp. 79–83). Wiley.

Ellis, A., & Harper, R. A. (1979). *A new guide to rational living* (Rev. Ed.). Wilshire Books.

Ellis, W. R., & Dietz, W. H. (2017). A new framework for addressing adverse childhood and community experiences: The building community resilience model. *Academic Pediatrics, 17*(7), S86–S93.

Epstein, J. N., & Loren, R. E. (2013). Changes in the definition of ADHD in DSM-5: Subtle but important. *Neuropsychiatry, 3*(5), 455.

Esser, M. B., Hedden, S. L., Kanny, D., Brewer, R. D., Gfroerer, J. C., & Naimi, T. S. (2014). Peer reviewed: Prevalence of alcohol dependence among US adult drinkers, 2009–2011. *Preventing Chronic Disease, 11*, e206. https://doi.org/10.5888/pcd11.140329

Esterson, A. (1998). Jeffrey Masson and Freud's seduction theory: A new fable based on old myths. *History of the Human Sciences, 11*(1), 1–21.

Eubanks, C. F., Goldfried, M. R., & Norcross, J. C. (2019). Future directions in psychotherapy integration. In J. C. Norcross & M. R. Goldfried (Eds.), *Handbook of psychotherapy integration* (3rd ed., pp. 474–85). Oxford Academic. https://doi.org/10.1093/med-psych/9780190690465.001.0001

Farrow, T. F., Hunter, M. D., Wilkinson, I. D., Gouneea, C., Fawbert, D., Smith, R., Lee, K. H., Mason, S., Spence, S. A., & Woodruff, P. W. (2005). Quantifiable change in functional brain response to empathic and forgivability judgments with resolution of posttraumatic stress disorder. *Psychiatry Research: Neuroimaging, 140*(1), 45–53. https://doi.org/10.1016/j.pscychresns.2005.05.012

Felitti, V. J., Anda, R. F., Nordenberg, D., & Williamson, D. F. (1998). Adverse childhood experiences and health outcomes in adults: The ACE study. *Journal of Family and Consumer Sciences, 90*(3), 31.

Felitti, V. J., Anda, R. F., Nordenberg, D., Williamson, D. F., Spitz, A. M., Edwards, V., Koss, M. P., & Marks, J. S. (2019). Relationship of childhood abuse and household dysfunction to many of the leading causes of death in adults: The adverse childhood experiences (ACE) study. *American Journal of Preventive Medicine, 56*(6), 774–786. https://doi.org/10.1016/j.amepre.2019.04.001

Figueiredo, T., Lima, G., Erthal, P., Martins, R., Corção, P., Leonel, M., Ayrão, V., Fortes, D., & Mattos, P. (2020). Mind-wandering, depression, anxiety and ADHD: Disentangling the relationship. *Psychiatry Research, 285*, 112798. https://doi.org/10.1016/j.psychres.2020.112798

Fils-Aime, L. (2021). To be anti-oppressive, CBT must consider identity. *Psychology Today*. https://www.psychologytoday.com/us/blog/the-gift-anti-racist-therapy/202109/be-anti-oppressive-cbt-must-consider-identity

Finlay, M., & Starmans, C. (2022). Not the same same: Distinguishing between similarity and identity in judgments of change. *Cognition, 218*, 104953. https://doi.org/10.1016/j.cognition.2021.104953

Fisher, A. J. (2015). Toward a dynamic model of psychological assessment: Implications for personalized care. *Journal of Consulting and Clinical Psychology, 83*(4), 825.

Fisher, A. J., Medaglia, J. D., & Jeronimus, B. F. (2018). Lack of group-to-individual generalizability is a threat to human subjects research. *Proceedings of the National Academy of Sciences, 115*(27), E6106–E6115.

Fitzgerald, M. H. (2000). Establishing cultural competency for mental health professionals. In J. Cox & V. Skultans (Eds.), *Anthropological Approaches to Psychological Medicine* (pp. 184–200). Jessica Kingsley.

Flückiger, C., Del Re, A. C., Wampold, B. E., & Horvath, A. O. (2018). The alliance in adult psychotherapy: A meta-analytic synthesis. *Psychotherapy, 55*(4), 316.

Fox, K. C., Andrews-Hanna, J. R., & Christoff, K. (2016). The neurobiology of self-generated thought from cells to systems: Integrating evidence from lesion studies, human intracranial electrophysiology, neurochemistry, and neuroendocrinology. *Neuroscience, 335*, 134–50.

Frances, A. (2013). *Saving normal: An insider's revolt against out-of-control psychiatric diagnosis, DSM-5, big pharma, and the medicalization of ordinary life.* HarperCollins.

Frankel, J. B. (1998). Ferenczi's trauma theory. *American Journal of Psychoanalysis, 58*(1), 41–61.

Frankl, V. E. (1985). *Man's search for meaning.* Simon and Schuster.

Franklin, B. (1998). *Autobiography and other writings.* Oxford University Press.

Freimuth, M. (2009). *Hidden addictions: Assessment practices for psychotherapists, counselors, and health care providers.* Jason Aronson.

Fromm, E. (1967). *The art of loving.* Bantam Books.

Gafori, H. L. (2022). Gold—Rumi. *New York Review of Books.*

Gay, P. (1998). *Freud: A life for our time.* W. W. Norton & Company.

Gazzaniga, M. (2011). *Who's in charge? Free will and the science of the brain.* HarperCollins.

George, D. A. (2021). *Unconscious bias: The prejudice of open-minded people (Diversity, inclusion and unconscious bias).* Independently published.

Gershon, M. (1999). *The second brain.* HarperPerennial.

Giacobbi, P. R. Jr., Stewart, J., Chaffee, K., Jaeschke, A. M., Stabler, M., & Kelley, G. A. (2017). A scoping review of health outcomes examined in randomized controlled trials using guided imagery. *Progress in Preventive Medicine, 2*(7), e0010.

Glasser, W. (1965). *Reality therapy: A new approach to psychiatry.* Harper & Row.

Goldfried, M. R. (2019). Obtaining consensus in psychotherapy: What holds us back? *American Psychologist, 74*(4), 484–496. https://doi.org/10.1037/amp0000365

Gollwitzer, P. M., & Sheeran, P. (2006). Implementation intentions and goal achievement: A meta-analysis of effects and processes. *Advances in Experimental Social Psychology, 38*, 69–119.

Greenberg, L. S. (2011). *Emotion-focused therapy.* American Psychological Association.

Greenwood, H., Krzyzaniak, N., Peiris, R., Clark, J., Scott, A. M., Cardona, M., Griffith, R., & Glasziou, P. (2022). Telehealth versus face-to-face psychotherapy for less common mental health conditions: Systematic review and meta-analysis of randomized controlled trials. *Journal of Medical Internet Research Mental Health, 9*(3), e31780.

Hacking, I. (1998). *Rewriting the soul.* Princeton University Press.

Hanh, T. N. (2017). *The art of living.* HarperCollins.

Hall, G. C. N., Berkman, E. T., Zane, N. W., Leong, F. T., Hwang, W. C., Nezu, A. M., Hong, J. J., Chu, J. J., & Huang, E. R. (2021). Reducing mental health disparities by increasing the personal relevance of interventions. *American Psychologist, 76*(1), 91–103. https://doi.org/10.1037/amp0000616

Haw, C., & Stubbs, J. (2007). Off-label use of antipsychotics: Are we mad? *Expert Opinion on Drug Safety, 6*(5), 533–545.

Hayes, S. C., with Smith, S. (2005). *Get out of your mind & into your life: The new acceptance and commitment therapy.* New Harbinger Publications.

Held, P., Smith, D. L., Pridgen, S., Coleman, J. A., & Klassen, B. J. (2023). More is not always better: 2 weeks of intensive cognitive processing therapy-based treatment are noninferior to 3 weeks. *Psychological Trauma: Theory, Research, Practice, and Policy, 15*(1), 100–109. https://doi.org/10.1037/tra0001257

Helms, J. E. (1994). How multiculturalism obscures racial factors in the therapy process: Comment on Ridley et al. (1994), Sodowsky et al. (1994), Ottavi et al. (1994), and Thompson et al. (1994). *Journal of Counseling Psychology, 41*(2), 162–165. https://doi.org/10.1037/0022-0167.41.2.162

Henson, C., Truchot, D., & Canevello, A. (2021). What promotes post traumatic growth? A systematic review. *European Journal of Trauma & Dissociation, 5*(4), 100195. https://doi.org/10.1016/j.ejtd.2020.100195

Herman, J. L. (1992). Complex PTSD: A syndrome in survivors of prolonged and repeated trauma. *Journal of Traumatic Stress, 5*(3), 377–391. https://doi.org/10.1002/jts.2490050305

Hilert, A. J., & Tirado, C. (2019). Teaching multicultural counseling with mindfulness: A contemplative pedagogy approach. *International Journal for the Advancement of Counselling, 41*, 469–480.

Hofmann, S. G., & Hayes, S. C. (2019). The future of intervention science: Process-based therapy. *Clinical Psychological Science, 7*(1), 37–50.

Hook, J. N. (2014). Engaging clients with cultural humility. *Journal of Psychology and Christianity, 33*(3), 277–281.

Hook, J. N., & Davis, D. E. (2019). Cultural humility: Introduction to the special issue. *Journal of Psychology and Theology, 47*(2), 71–75.

Hook, J. N., Farrell, J. E., Davis, D. E., DeBlaere, C., Van Tongeren, D. R., & Utsey, S. O. (2016). Cultural humility and racial microaggressions in counseling. *Journal of Counseling Psychology, 63*(3), 269.

Hor, C. N., Yeung, J., Jan, M., Emmenegger, Y., Hubbard, J., Xenarios, I., Naef, F., & Franken, P. (2019). Sleep–wake-driven and circadian contributions to daily rhythms in gene expression and chromatin accessibility in the murine cortex. *Proceedings of the National Academy of Sciences, 116*(51), 25773–25783. https://doi.org/10.1073/pnas.1910590116

Horney, K. (1950, 1991). *Neurosis and human growth: The struggle toward self-realization* (Vol. 10). Norton.

Hurley, W. C. (2021). *Compassion's compass: Strategies for developing insight, kindness, and empathy.* Rowman & Littlefield.

International Buddhist Information and Research Center (IBIRC). (1993). *The path to inner peace and happiness: Selected verses from the Dhammapada and other sayings of the Buddha.* Buddhist Centre Toronto Maravihara.

James, W. (1900). *Talks to teachers and students.* Holt.

Janis, R. A., Burlingame, G. M., Svien, H., Jensen, J., & Lundgreen, R. (2021). Group therapy for mood disorders: A meta-analysis. *Psychotherapy Research, 31*(3), 342–358.

Jaspers, J. P. C. (2003). Lumpers versus splitters. *Journal of Psychosomatic Obstetrics & Gynecology, 24*(4), 213–214.

Kagan, J., Arcus, D., Snidman, N., Feng, W. Y., Hendler, J., & Greene, S. (1994). Reactivity in infants: A cross-national comparison. *Developmental Psychology, 30*(3), 342.

Kagan, J., & Snidman, N. (1999). Early childhood predictors of adult anxiety disorders. *Biological Psychiatry, 46*(11), 1536–1541.

Kaldo, V., Bothelius, K., Blom, K., Lindhe, M., Larsson, M., Karimi, K., Melder, S., Bondestam, V., Ulfsparre, C., Sternbrink, K., & Jernelöv, S. (2020). An open-ended primary-care group intervention for insomnia based on a self-help book—A randomized controlled trial and 4-year follow-up. *Journal of Sleep Research, 29*(1), e12881.

Kamiya, K., Fumoto, M., Kikuchi, H., Sekiyama, T., Mohri-Ikuzawa, Y., Umino, M., & Arita, H. (2010). Prolonged gum chewing evokes activation of the ventral part of prefrontal cortex and suppression of nociceptive responses: Involvement of the serotonergic system. *Journal of Medical and Dental Sciences, 57*(1), 35–43.

Kazantzis, N., Whittington, C., Zelencich, L., Kyrios, M., Norton, P. J., & Hofmann, S. G. (2016). Quantity and quality of homework compliance: A meta-analysis of relations with outcome in cognitive behavior therapy. *Behavior Therapy, 47*(5), 755–772.

Kellam, S. G., Mackenzie, A. C., Brown, C. H., Poduska, J. M., Wang, W., Petras, H., & Wilcox, H. C. (2011). The good behavior game and the future of prevention and treatment. *Addiction Science & Clinical Practice, 6*(1), 73.

Kellogg, S. (1993). Identity and recovery. *Psychotherapy: Theory, Research, Practice, Training, 30*(2), 235.

Kellogg, S. (2014). *Transformational chairwork: Using psychotherapeutic dialogues in clinical practice.* Rowman & Littlefield.

Kelso, J. S. (2012). Multistability and metastability: understanding dynamic coordination in the brain. *Philosophical Transactions of the Royal Society B: Biological Sciences, 367*(1591), 906–918.

Kent, S. T., McClure, L. A., Crosson, W. L., Arnett, D. K., Wadley, V. G., & Sathiakumar, N. (2009). Effect of sunlight exposure on cognitive function among depressed and non-depressed participants: A REGARDS cross-sectional study. *Environmental Health, 8*(1), 1–14.

Killingsworth, M. A., & Gilbert, D. T. (2010). A wandering mind is an unhappy mind. *Science, 330*(6006), 932. https://doi.org/10.1126/science.1192439

Korzybski, A. (1958). *Science and sanity: An introduction to non-Aristotelian systems and general semantics.* Institute of General Semantics.

Koshimori, Y. (2019). Neurochemical responses to music. In M. H. Thaut & D. A. Hodges (Eds.), *The Oxford handbook of music and the brain* (pp. 333–363). Oxford University Press.

Koshimori, Y., & Thaut, M. H. (2019). New perspectives on music in rehabilitation of executive and attention functions. *Frontiers in Neuroscience, 13*, 1245.

Kraus, D. R., Castonguay, L., Boswell, J. F., Nordberg, S. S., & Hayes, J. A. (2011). Therapist effectiveness: Implications for accountability and patient care. *Psychotherapy Research, 21*(3), 267–276.

Krebs, P., Norcross, J. C., Nicholson, J. M., & Prochaska, J. O. (2018). Stages of change and psychotherapy outcomes: A review and meta-analysis. *Journal of Clinical Psychology, 74*(11), 1964–1979.

Kringelbach, M. L., & Berridge, K. C. (2017). The affective core of emotion: Linking pleasure, subjective well-being, and optimal metastability in the brain. *Emotion Review, 9*(3), 191–199.

Krizan, Z., & Hisler, G. (2019). Sleepy anger: Restricted sleep amplifies angry feelings. *Journal of Experimental Psychology: General, 148*(7), 1239.

Krzyzaniak, N., Greenwood, H., Scott, A. M., Peiris, R., Cardona, M., Clark, J., & Glasziou, P. (2021). The effectiveness of telehealth versus face-to face interventions for anxiety disorders: A systematic review and meta-analysis. *Journal of Telemedicine and Telecare,* 1357633X211053738. https://doi.org/10.1177/1357633X211053738

Lazarus, A. A. (1981). *The practice of multimodal therapy.* McGraw-Hill.

Leake, G. J., & King, A. S. (1977). Effect of counselor expectations on alcoholic recovery. *Alcohol Health & Research World, 1*(3), 16–22.

Lefevor, G. T., Goldblum, P., Dowling, K. T., Goodman, J. A., Hoeflein, B., & Skidmore, S. J. (2022). First do no harm: Principles of care for clients with sexual identity confusion and/or conflict. *Psychotherapy, 59*(4), 487–497. https://doi.org/10.1037/pst0000426.

Leifer, R. (2008). *Vinegar into honey: Seven steps to understanding and transforming anger, aggression, and violence.* Shambhala Publications.

Leopold, S. S. (2021). A conversation with . . . Ted. J. Kaptchuk, expert in placebo effects. *Clinical Orthopaedics and Related Research, 479*(8), 1645–1650.

Lewis-Fernández, R., Aggarwal, N. K., & Kirmayer, L. J. (2020). The cultural formulation Interview: Progress to date and future directions. *Transcultural Psychiatry, 57*(4), 487–496.

Liese, B. S., & Esterline, K. M. (2015). Concept mapping: A supervision strategy for introducing case conceptualization skills to novice therapists. *Psychotherapy, 52*(2), 190.

Lilienfeld, S. O. (2007). Psychological treatments that cause harm. *Perspectives on Psychological Science, 2*(1), 53–70.

Linehan, M. (2014). *DBT Skills training manual.* Guilford Publications.

Linehan, M. M. (2018). *Cognitive-behavioral treatment of borderline personality disorder.* Guilford Publications.

Linehan, M. M., Armstrong, H. E., Suarez, A., Allmon, D., & Heard, H. L. (1991). Cognitive-behavioral treatment of chronically parasuicidal borderline patients. *Archives of General Psychiatry, 48*(12), 1060–1064.

Lopez-Quintero, C., Hasin, D. S., De Los Cobos, J. P., Pines, A., Wang, S., Grant, B. F., & Blanco, C. (2011). Probability and predictors of remission from life-time nicotine, alcohol, cannabis or cocaine dependence: Results from the national epidemiologic survey on alcohol and related conditions. *Addiction, 106*(3), 657–669.

Maguire, E. A., Gadian, D. G., Johnsrude, I. S., Good, C. D., Ashburner, J., Frackowiak, R. S., & Frith, C. D. (2000). Navigation-related structural change in the hippocampi of taxi drivers. *Proceedings of the National Academy of Sciences, 97*(8), 4398–4403.

Maguire, E. A., Woollett, K., & Spiers, H. J. (2006). London taxi drivers and bus drivers: A structural MRI and neuropsychological analysis. *Hippocampus, 16*(12), 1091–1101.

Malhotra, S., & Sahoo, S. (2017). Rebuilding the brain with psychotherapy. *Indian Journal of Psychiatry, 59*(4), 411.

Marcelin, J. R., Siraj, D. S., Victor, R., Kotadia, S., & Maldonado, Y. A. (2019). The impact of unconscious bias in healthcare: How to recognize and mitigate it. *Journal of Infectious Diseases, 220*(Supplement_2), S62–S73. https://doi.org/10.1093/infdis/jiz214

Marlatt, A., & Gordon, J. (1985). *Relapse prevention: Maintenance strategies in the treatment of addictive behaviors.* Guilford.

Mason, L., Peters, E., Williams, S. C., & Kumari, V. (2017). Brain connectivity changes occurring following cognitive behavioural therapy for psychosis predict long-term recovery. *Translational Psychiatry, 7*(1), e1001–e1001.

Masson, J. M. (2012). *The assault on truth*. Untreed Reads.

Mausbach, B. T., Moore, R., Roesch, S., Cardenas, V., & Patterson, T. L. (2010). The relationship between homework compliance and therapy outcomes: An updated meta-analysis. *Cognitive Therapy and Research, 34*, 429–438.

Maultsby, M. (1971). Rational emotive imagery. *Rational Living, 6*(1), 24–27.

May, R. (1969, 2007). *Love and will*. Norton.

McCrary, J. M., Redding, E., & Altenmüller, E. (2021). Performing arts as a health resource? An umbrella review of the health impacts of music and dance participation. *PloS ONE, 16*(6), e0252956.

McCullough, M. L. (2001). Freud's seduction theory and its rehabilitation: A saga of one mistake after another. *Review of General Psychology, 5*(1), 3–22.

McDonald, M., Brandt, M., & Bluhm, R. (2017). From shell-shock to PTSD, a century of invisible war trauma. *The Conversation, 4*.

Meechan, C. F., Laws, K. R., Young, A. H., McLoughlin, D. M., & Jauhar, S. (2022). A critique of narrative reviews of the evidence-base for ECT in depression. *Epidemiology and Psychiatric Sciences, 31*. https://doi.org/10.1017/S2045796021000731

Meng, M., Lv, M., Wang, L., Yang, B., Jiao, P., Lei, W., Lan, H., Shen, Q., Luo, X., Yu, X., Xun, Y., Leu, R., Hou, T., Chen, Y., & Li, Q. (2022). Off-label use of drugs in pediatrics: A scoping review. *European Journal of Pediatrics*, 1–11. https://doi.org/10.1007/s00431-022-04515-7

Miller, W. R. (2004). The phenomenon of quantum change. *Journal of Clinical Psychology, 60*(5), 453–460.

Miller, W. R. & Rollnick, S. (2012). *Motivational interviewing: Helping people change*. Guilford Press.

Miller, W. T. (1995). Increasing motivation for change. In R. K. Hester & W. R. Miller (Eds.), *Alcoholism treatment approaches: Effective approaches (2nd ed.)* (pp. 89–014). Allyn & Bacon.

Mischel, W. (2008). The toothbrush problem. *APS Observer, 21*.

Mishra, A., Chaturvedi, P., Datta, S., Sinukumar, S., Joshi, P., & Garg, A. (2015). Harmful effects of nicotine. *Indian Journal of Medical and Paediatric Oncology, 36*(01), 24–31.

Mlodinow, L. (2009). *The drunkard's walk: How randomness rules our lives*. Vintage.

Mollen, D., & Ridley, C. R. (2021). Rethinking multicultural counseling competence: An introduction to the major contribution. *Counseling Psychologist, 49*(4), 490–503.

Moncrieff, J. (2006). Why is it so difficult to stop psychiatric drug treatment? It may be nothing to do with the original problem. *Medical Hypotheses, 67*(3), 517–523.

Montesano, A., Feixas, G., Caspar, F., & Winter, D. (2017). Depression and identity: Are self-constructions negative or conflictual? *Frontiers in Psychology, 8*, 877.

Mosini, A. C., Saad, M., Braghetta, C. C., Medeiros, R. D., Peres, M. F. P., & Leão, F. C. (2019). Neurophysiological, cognitive-behavioral and neurochemical effects in practitioners of transcendental meditation: A literature review. *Revista da Associação Médica Brasileira*, 65, 706–713.

Moyers, T. B., & Miller, W. R. (2013). Is low therapist empathy toxic? *Psychology of Addictive Behaviors, 27*(3), 878.

Murphy, C. M., Eckhardt, C. I., Clifford, J. M., LaMotte, A. D., & Meis, L. A. (2020). Individual versus group cognitive-behavioral therapy for partner-violent men: A preliminary randomized trial. *Journal of Interpersonal Violence, 35*(15–16), 2846–2868.

Narayanan, S., & Terris, E. (2020). Inclusive manufacturing: The impact of disability diversity on productivity in a work integration social enterprise. *Manufacturing & Service Operations Management, 22*(6), 1112–1130.

Nauphal, M., Swetlitz, C., Smith, L., & Rosellini, A. J. (2021). A preliminary examination of the acceptability, feasibility, and effectiveness of a telehealth cognitive-behavioral therapy group for social anxiety disorder. *Cognitive and Behavioral Practice, 28*(4), 730–742.

Neff, G., & Nafus, D. (2016). *Self-tracking*. MIT Press.

Nolan, J. D., Houlihan, D., Wanzek, M., & Jenson, W. R. (2014). The good behavior game: A classroom-behavior intervention effective across cultures. *School Psychology International, 35*(2), 191–205.

Norcross, J. C., & Goldfried, M. R. (Eds.). (2005). *Handbook of psychotherapy integration.* Oxford University Press.

Norcross, J. C., & Lambert, M. J. (2018). Psychotherapy relationships that work III. *Psychotherapy, 55*(4), 303.

Norcross, J. C., & Wampold, B. E. (2018). A new therapy for each patient: Evidence-based relationships and responsiveness. *Journal of Clinical Psychology, 74*(11), 1889–1906.

Nordell, J. (2021). *The end of bias: A beginning: The science and practice of overcoming unconscious bias.* Metropolitan Books.

Norwood, C., Moghaddam, N. G., Malins, S., & Sabin-Farrell, R. (2018). Working alliance and outcome effectiveness in videoconferencing psychotherapy: A systematic review and noninferiority meta-analysis. *Clinical Psychology & Psychotherapy, 25*(6), 797–808.

Ogle, C. M., Rubin, D. C., Berntsen, D., & Siegler, I. C. (2013). The frequency and impact of exposure to potentially traumatic events over the life course. *Clinical Psychological Science, 1*(4), 426–434.

Padesky, C. A. (1989). Attaining and maintaining positive lesbian self-identity: A cognitive therapy approach. *Women & Therapy, 8*(1–2), 145–156. https://doi.org/10.1300/J015v08n01_12

Padesky, C. A. (2020). Collaborative case conceptualization: Client knows best. *Cognitive and Behavioral Practice, 27*(4), 392–404.

Pandi-Perumal, S. R., Monti, J. M., Burman, D., Karthikeyan, R., BaHammam, A. S., Spence, D. W., Brown, G. M., & Narashimhan, M. (2020). Clarifying the role of sleep in depression: A narrative review. *Psychiatry Research, 291*, 113239. 10.1016/j.psychres.2020.113239

Perls, F. S. (1969). *Gestalt therapy verbatim.* Real People Press.

Persons, J. B. (2012). *The case formulation approach to cognitive-behavior therapy.* Guilford.

Peterson, A. L., Mintz, J., Moring, J. C., Straud, C. L., Young-McCaughan, S., McGeary, C. A., McGeary, D. D., Litz, B. T., Velligan, D. I., Macdonald, A., Mata-Galan, E., Holliday, S. L., Dillon, K. H., Roache, J. D., Bira, L. M., Nabity, P. S., Medellin, E. M., Hale, W. J., & Resick, P. A. (2022). In-office, in-home, and telehealth cognitive processing therapy for posttraumatic stress disorder in veterans: A randomized clinical trial. *BMC Psychiatry, 22*(1), 41. https://doi.org/10.1186/s12888-022-03699-4

Porges, S. W. (2011). *The polyvagal theory: Neurophysiological foundations of emotions, attachment, communication, and self-regulation.* Norton.

Prochaska, J. O., & DiClemente, C. C. (1982). Transtheoretical therapy: Toward a more integrative model of change. *Psychotherapy: Theory, Research & Practice, 19*(3), 276–288. https://doi.org/10.1037/h0088437

Prochaska, J. O., DiClemente, C. C., & Norcross, J. (1992). In search of how people change. *American Psychologist, 47*(9), 1101–1114.

Prochnik, G. (2012). *Putnam camp: Sigmund Freud, James Jackson Putnam and the purpose of American psychology.* Other Press.

Read, J., Kirsch, I., & McGrath, L. (2020). Electroconvulsive therapy for depression: A review of the quality of ECT versus sham ECT trials and meta-analyses. *BJPsych Advances, 27*(5), 284. https://doi.org/10.1192/bja.2021.25

Resick, P. A., Monson, C. M., & Chard, K. M. (2016). *Cognitive processing therapy for PTSD: A comprehensive manual.* Guilford Publications.

Resick, P. A., Wachen, J. S., Dondanville, K. A., Pruiksma, K. E., Yarvis, J. S., Peterson, A. L., Mintz, J., Strong Star Consortium, Borah, E. V., Brundige, A., Hembree, E. A., Litz, B. T., Roache, J. D., & Young-McCaughan, S. (2017). Effect of group vs individual cognitive processing therapy in active-duty military seeking treatment for posttraumatic stress disorder: A randomized clinical trial. *JAMA Psychiatry, 74*(1), 28–36. https://doi.org/10.1001/jamapsychiatry.2016.2729

Ridley, C. R., Mendoza, D. W., & Kanitz, B. E. (1994). Multicultural training: Reexamination, operationalization, and integration. *Counseling Psychologist, 22*(2), 227–289.

Ridley, C. R., Sahu, A., Console, K., Surya, S., Tran, V., Xie, S., & Yin, C. (2021). The process model of multicultural counseling competence. *Counseling Psychologist, 49*(4), 534–567.

Robb, H. (2022), *Willingly ACT for spiritual development: Acknowledge, choose, & teach others.* Independently published.

Roberts, B. W., & Mroczek, D. (2008). Personality trait change in adulthood. *Current Directions in Psychological Science, 17*(1), 31–35.

Rogers, C. R. (1951). *Client-centered therapy: Its current practice, implications and theory.* Houghton Mifflin.

Rogers, C. R. (1957). The necessary and sufficient conditions of therapeutic personality change. *Journal of Consulting Psychology, 21*(2), 95.

Rosa, R. R., Bonnet, M. H., & Kramer, M. (1983). The relationship of sleep and anxiety in anxious subjects. *Biological Psychology, 16*(1–2), 119–126.

Saks, E. R. (2013, January 25). Successful and schizophrenic. *New York Times.*

Schwartz, J. M. (1996). *Brain lock: Free yourself from obsessive-compulsive behavior.* HarperCollins.

Scott, A. M., Bakhit, M., Greenwood, H., Cardona, M., Clark, J., Krzyzaniak, N., Peiris, R., & Glasziou, P. (2022). Real-time telehealth versus face-to-face management for patients with PTSD in primary care: A systematic review and meta-analysis. *Journal of Clinical Psychiatry, 83*(4), 41146.

Shao, M., Lin, X., Jiang, D., Tian, H., Xu, Y., Wang, L., Ji, F., Zhou, C., Song, X., & Zhuo, C. (2020). Depression and cardiovascular disease: Shared molecular mechanisms and clinical implications. *Psychiatry Research, 285*, 112802. https://doi.org/10.1016/j.psychres.2020.112802

Sheikh, A. A. (2020). *Handbook of therapeutic imagery techniques.* Routledge.

Singh, R. S., Bhambhani, Y., Skinta, M. D., & Torres-Harding, S. R. (2021). Measurement of intersectional microaggressions: Conceptual barriers and recommendations. *Perspectives on Psychological Science, 16*(5), 956–971. https://journals.sagepub.com/doi/full/10.1177/1745691621991855

Skottnik, L., & Linden, D. E. (2019). Mental imagery and brain regulation—New links between psychotherapy and neuroscience. *Frontiers in Psychiatry, 10*, 779.

Soares, W. E. III, Knowles, K. J., & Friedmann, P. D. (2019). A thousand cuts: Racial and ethnic disparities in emergency medicine. *Medical Care, 57*(12), 921.

Sollod, R. N. (2005). Integrating spirituality with psychotherapy. In J. C. Norcross & M. R. Goldfried (Eds.), *Handbook of psychotherapy integration* (3rd ed., pp. 405–431). Oxford University Press. https://doi.org/10.1093/med:psych/9780195165791.003.0019

Somer, E., Cardeña, E., Catelan, R. F., & Soffer-Dudek, N. (2021). Reality shifting: Psychological features of an emergent online daydreaming culture. *Current Psychology, 42*, 1–13. https://doi.org/10.1007/s12144-021-02439-3

Sonmez, A. I., Camsari, D. D., Nandakumar, A. L., Voort, J. L. V., Kung, S., Lewis, C. P., & Croarkin, P. E. (2019). Accelerated TMS for depression: A systematic review and meta-analysis. *Psychiatry Research, 273*, 770–781.

Spielmans, I. G. (2015). Atypical antipsychotics: Overrated and overprescribed. *Pharmaceutical Journal, 294*, 7851.

Stapleton, S. M., Bababekov, Y. J., Perez, N. P., Fong, Z. V., Hashimoto, D. A., Lillemoe, K. D., Watkins, M. T., & Chang, D. C. (2018). Variation in amputation risk for black patients: Uncovering potential sources of bias and opportunities for intervention. *Journal of the American College of Surgeons, 226*(4), 641–649.

Steiger, V. R., Brühl, A. B., Weidt, S., Delsignore, A., Rufer, M., Jäncke, L., Herwig, U., & Hänggi, J. (2017). Pattern of structural brain changes in social anxiety disorder after cognitive behavioral group therapy: A longitudinal multimodal MRI study. *Molecular Psychiatry, 22*(8), 1164–1171.

Stewart, R. W., Orengo-Aguayo, R., Young, J., Wallace, M. M., Cohen, J. A., Mannarino, A. P., & de Arellano, M. A. (2020). Feasibility and effectiveness of a telehealth service delivery model for treating childhood posttraumatic stress: A community-based, open pilot trial of trauma-focused cognitive–behavioral therapy. *Journal of Psychotherapy Integration, 30*(2), 274–289. https://doi.org/10.1037/int0000225

Stirman, S. W., Song, J., Hull, T. D., & Resick, P. A. (2021). Open trial of an adaptation of cognitive processing therapy for message-based delivery. *Technology, Mind, and Behavior, 2*(1). https://doi.org /10.1037/tmb0000016

Stover, C. S., Hahn, H., Maciejewski, K. R., Epstein, C., & Marans, S. (2022). The child and family traumatic stress intervention: Factors associated with symptom reduction for children receiving treatment. *Child Abuse & Neglect, 134*, 105886.

Sue, D. W., Capodilupo, C. M., Torino, G. C., Bucceri, J. M., Holder, A., Nadal, K. L., & Esquilin, M. (2007). Racial microaggressions in everyday life: Implications for clinical practice. *American Psychologist, 62*(4), 271.

Takahashi, T., Kikai, T., Sugiyama, F., Kawashima, I., Kuroda, A., Usui, K., Maeda, W., Uchida, T., Guan, S., Oguchi, M., & Kumano, H. (2020). Changes in mind-wandering and cognitive fusion through mindfulness group therapy for depression and anxiety. *Journal of Cognitive Psychotherapy, 34*(2). https://doi.org/10.1891/JCPSY-D-19-00015

Tengeler, A. C., Dam, S. A., Wiesmann, M., Naaijen, J., Van Bodegom, M., Belzer, C., Dederen, P. J., Verweij, V., Franke, B., Kozicz, T., Vasquez, A. A., & Kiliaan, A. J. (2020). Gut microbiota from persons with attention-deficit/hyperactivity disorder affects the brain in mice. *Microbiome, 8*, 1–14.

Tolman, E. C. (1951). *Purposive behavior in animals and men.* University of California Press.

van der Kolk, B. (2014). *The Body keeps the score: Brain, mind, and body in the healing of trauma.* Penguin.

Vandiver, B. J., Delgado-Romero, E. A., & Liu, W. M. (2021). Is multicultural counseling competence outdated or underdeveloped, or in need of refinement? A response to Ridley et al. *Counseling Psychologist, 49*(4), 586–609.

Vicedo, M. (2020). Attachment theory from ethology to the strange situation. In W. E. Pickren (Ed.), *Oxford research encyclopedia of psychology.* https://doi.org/10.1093/acrefore/9780190236557.013 .524

Watters, E. (2010). *Crazy like us: The globalization of the American psyche.* Simon & Schuster.

Welz, A., Reinhard, I., Alpers, G., & Kuehner, C. (2018). Happy thoughts: Mind wandering affects mood in daily life. *Mindfulness, 9*(1), 332–343. https://doi.org/10.1007/s12671-017-0778-y

West, R. (2005). Time for a change: Putting the transtheoretical (stages of change) model to rest [Editorial]. *Addiction, 100*(8), 1036–1039. https://doi.org/10.1111/j.1360-0443.2005.01139.x

West, R., & Brown, J. (2013). *Theory of addiction.* Wiley.

Wilcox, H. C., Kellam, S. G., Brown, C. H., Poduska, J. M., Ialongo, N. S., Wang, W., & Anthony, J. C. (2008). The impact of two universal randomized first- and second-grade classroom interventions on young adult suicide ideation and attempts. *Drug and Alcohol Dependence, 95*, S60–S73.

Wilson, E. (2018). *Homer: The odyssey.* Norton.

Wong, Y. L. R., & Vinsky, J. (2021). Beyond implicit bias: Embodied cognition, mindfulness, and critical reflective practice in social work. *Australian Social Work, 74*(2), 186–197.

Woon, F. L., Sood, S., & Hedges, D. W. (2010). Hippocampal volume deficits associated with exposure to psychological trauma and posttraumatic stress disorder in adults: A meta-analysis. *Progress in Neuro-Psychopharmacology and Biological Psychiatry, 34*(7), 1181–1188.

Xu, H., & Zhuang, X. (2019). Atypical antipsychotics-induced metabolic syndrome and nonalcoholic fatty liver disease: A critical review. *Neuropsychiatric Disease and Treatment*, 2087–2099. https://doi .org/10.2147/NDT.S208061

Zanarini, M. C., Frankenburg, F. R., Reich, D. B., & Fitzmaurice, G. (2010). Time to attainment of recovery from borderline personality disorder and stability of recovery: A 10-year prospective follow-up study. *American Journal of Psychiatry, 167*(6), 663–667.

Zhang, H., Watkins, C. E. Jr., Hook, J. N., Hodge, A. S., Davis, C. W., Norton, J., Wilcox, M. M., Davis, D. E., DeBlaere, C., & Owen, J. (2022). Cultural humility in psychotherapy and clinical supervision: A research review. *Counselling and Psychotherapy Research, 22*(3), 548–557.

Zheng, P., Zeng, B., Zhou, C., Liu, M., Fang, Z., Xu, X., Zeng, L., Chen, J., Fan, S., Du, X., Zhang, X., Yang, D., Yang, Y., Meng, H., Li, W., Melgiri, N. D., Licinio, J., Wei, H., & Xie, P. (2016). Gut microbiome remodeling induces depressive-like behaviors through a pathway mediated by the host's metabolism. *Molecular Psychiatry, 21*(6), 786–796.

Index

AAPs. *See* atypical antipsychotics
ABC(DE) exercises, vii; activating event, 52; beliefs about activating event, 52–53; between-session work and, 65, 67; coaching and, 160; consequences of, 52–53; disputing, 53–54; effective thoughts, 54–55; in initial assessment, 29, 31; for in-session work, 51–55
acceptance, 116; mindfulness and, 88–91; neuroplasticity and, 114–15; over-emoting and, 97–98; under-emoting and, 97
acceptance and commitment therapy (ACT), 1, 20; "Attending Your Own Funeral" exercise, 70; in-session work and, 55
ACE study. *See* adverse childhood events study
ACT. *See* acceptance and commitment therapy
action stage, in Stages of Change model, 10
active listening, 25; with diverse clients, 75
ADA. *See* Americans with Disabilities Act
addiction behaviors, methodological approach to, 5
ADHD. *See* attention deficit and hyperactivity disorder
Adler, Albert, first three memories exercise, 129–30
Adlerian therapy, 1
adverse childhood events study (ACE study), 13, 124–25; diverse clients and, 71; existential influences on, 43; poverty influences in, 71–72; spiritual influences on, 43
agenda setting, for therapy, 47–48, 86
Albert Ellis Institute, 35
alcohol abuse and misuse: in *DMS-III*, 15; genetic inheritance of, 111; high alcohol recovery persons, 21; initial assessment of, 37; protective behavioral strategies for, 121; Stages of Change model for, 37
all-or-nothing thinking, 136
American Pain Society, 42–43
Americans with Disabilities Act (ADA), 72–73
analysis. *See* psychoanalysis; transactional analysis
anger management: initial assessment of, 31; protective behavioral strategies for, 121
Antabuse, 167
antisocial personality disorder, 66
anxiety disorders: genetic inheritance of, 111; protective behavioral strategies for, 121
The Art of Loving (Fromm), 99
assessment, initial: ABC(DE) exercises, 29, 31; of alcohol abuse, 37; of anger management, 31; BASIC-ID assessment approach, 30; case conceptualization in, 31–32; by clinicians, 34; cognitive behavioral therapy and, 31–32; Colombo technique and, 35–36; cultural formulation interview, 34; for depression, 35–36; *DSM-V* and, 32–33; ethics in, 33–34; harm minimization in, 33–34; for hidden addictions, 36; *ICD-10* and, 32–33; instruments for, 30; insurance and, 34; for marital counseling, 34; NOS assessment, 32; through previous assessments, 34; with PRIME model, 32–33; by researchers, 34; small talk as part of, 30; Stages of Change assessments, 30–31; structure of, 29; transdiagnostic approaches, 33; by type of therapy, 34–35

Atomic Habits (Clear), 152–53
attachment-based therapy, 1
attachment theory, 13
"Attending Your Own Funeral" exercise, 70
attention deficit and hyperactivity disorder (ADHD): as behavioral problem, viii; between-session work with, 66; blaming with, 112; genetic inheritance and, 111–12; medications for, 164–65; shaming behaviors, 112
atypical antipsychotics (AAPs), 166
autobiographies, 120

BASIC-ID assessment approach, 30
Bateson, Gregory, 22
Beck, Aaron, 31. *See also* cognitive behavioral therapy; cognitive therapy
Beck Anxiety Scale, 30
Beck Depression Scale, 30
Beck Hopelessness Scale, 30
behavioral activation therapy, 1
behavioral storms, 15–16
behavior therapy (BT), 1
beliefs: in ABC(DE) exercises, 52–53; disputing irrational beliefs, 136–37; flexibility of, 53; helpful/rational, 53; in-session work and, 55, 57; unhelpful/irrational, 53, 119–20, 136–37
benzodiazepines, 59
between-session work: ABC(DE) exercises and, 65, 67; affirmation of client strengths, 65–66; alternative strategies for, 140; for antisocial personality disorder, 66; "Attending Your Own Funeral" exercise, 70; with attention deficit and hyperactivity disorder, 66; bibliotherapy and, 140–41; checking in, 135, 140; client exhaustion and, 85; client successes, 84; client task failure, 83–84; with cognitive behavioral therapy, 63; cost-benefit analysis of, 65, 122; disputing irrational beliefs, 136–37; exercise during, 70; as homework, viii, 82–83; identification of cognitive distortions, 63; key objectives of, 61; meditation and, 62–63; negative feedback loops, 67; for panic attacks, 66–67; for peer rejection anxiety, 66; prayer during, 62–63; radical acceptance strategies and, 140; reduction in suicide attempts, 66; reduction of experiential avoidance, 64–65; restarting previously successful approach, 62; risk-taking exercises, 63–64; school-based services, 66; self-maintenance/chores for, *138–39*; sleep habits and, 69–70; smartphones and, 69–70; Stages of Change model and, 61; take-home therapy exercises, 65; three-column technique, 138–39; value clarification exercises, 139–40; wearable technology and, 69–70
Bhikku, Thanissaro, 146
bibliotherapy, 59; between-session work and, 140–41
bioenergetics, 1
bipolar disorder: case studies, 26–27; Depakote treatment, 165; genetic inheritance of, 111; rational emotive behavior therapy with, 26
blaming: attention deficit and hyperactivity disorder and, 112; in-session work and, 50; rejection of, 74
The Body Keeps the Score (van der Kolk), 115
body work, 59
The Book of Joy (Dalai Lama and Tutu), 62–63, 93
borderline personality disorder (BPD), 149
Botton, Alain de, 44
box breathing, 58. *See also* deep diaphragmatic breathing
BPD. *See* borderline personality disorder
Bradshaw, John, 100
brain development, 114; transcendental self and, 115–16. *See also* neural modular networks
brain disease model, in psychotherapy, viii
"brain lies," 50–51
breathing exercises: box breathing, 58; deep diaphragmatic breathing, 8, 58–59
brief psychodynamic therapy, 1
brief relational therapy, 1
Bright-Sided (Ehrenreich), 98
Bronson, Po, 120
Brown, Laura, 151
Bruce, Lenny, 11
BT. *See* behavior therapy
Buchanan, Mark, 15
Buddha, 72, 87
Buddhism: for Ellis, 19; the self and, 146
Buddhism (Conze), 72
building a practice, 173; social networking, 174
bupropion, 168
burnout, 175–76; for counselors, 21

CALM app, 63, 103
CBA. *See* cost-benefit analysis
CBT. *See* cognitive behavioral therapy
CFT. *See* compassion-focused therapy
CFTSI. *See* Child and Family Traumatic Stress Intervention

chairwork, 106; expression of feelings through, 107

change behaviors: flash crash, 118; frequency, duration, and intensity approach to, 118; neuroplasticity and, 114–15. *See also* Stages of Change model

change talk, 25

Chantix. *See* varenicline

character, personality compared to, 147, 149

Charcot, Jean-Marie, 124

Child and Family Traumatic Stress Intervention (CFTSI), 127

Christianity, 11

classism, 151–52, 156

Clear, James, 152–53

client-centered therapy, 1, 47

clients: counselor friendships with, 23; diverse, 71–77; exhaustion of, 85; harmful questioning by, 156; identification and labeling of feelings, 98–99; identities for, 146–47; inner criticism, 154; motivation for therapy for, 20; self-confidence strategies, 153–54; self-criticism, 156. *See also* client-centered therapy; relationship with clients

clinicians, counselors and: burnout, 175–76; expectations of clients, 21; friendship with clients, 23; protections for, 174–75; self-care for, 21; self-disclosures by, 21, 27–28; self-reflection for, 73–74; transference between client and, 27; unhelpful protections for, 174–75

closed-ended questions, 25

coaching: ABC techniques, 160; discovery method, 157; executive, 161; life, 161; role-playing and, 160; slow discussions and, 159–60; therapeutic approaches compared to, 157–59

cognitive behavioral therapy (CBT), 1; between-session work with, 63; diverse clients and, 72; Ellis and, vii, 11–12; historical development of, 11; imagery use in, 100, 102–3; initial assessment and, 31–32; rational emotive therapy, vii, 11; Stoicism and, 11; transdiagnostic, 2; Veterans Administration program, 30

cognitive defusion techniques, motivational interviewing and, 120

cognitive distortions: identification of, 63; types of, 134–35

cognitive processing therapy (CPT), 1; for post-traumatic stress disorder, 126–27; "stuck points" in, 126–27

Cognitive Processing Therapy for PTSD (Resick), 126

Cognitive Psychology (Neisser), 11

cognitive therapy (CT), 1, 31

collaboration, collaborative approaches and, in psychotherapy, viii, 7; compliance as part of, 8; deep diaphragmatic breathing, 8; eclectic approaches, 8–9; integration of approaches from other cultures, 9–16; nomothetic approaches, 8; resistance to, 8; for session structure, 9

Columbo technique, 35–36; mindfulness and, 94–96

combined therapies, 171–72

compassion: mindfulness and, 98; self, 116

compassion-focused therapy (CFT), 1

Compassion's Compass (Hurley), 63

complex post-traumatic stress disorder (CPTSD), 125–26, 128

conditioning, in PRIME theory, 12

consultation approaches, therapy compared to, for diverse clients, 77

contemplation stage, in Stages of Change model, 10

Conze, Edward, 72

Cost-benefit analysis (CBA), of between-session work, 65, 122

counselors. *See* clinicians

COVID-19 pandemic, 179–80

CPT. *See* cognitive processing therapy

CPTSD. *See* complex post-traumatic stress disorder

Crazy Like Us (Watters), 71

CT. *See* cognitive therapy

Cuban, Mark, 91

cultural formulation interview, 34

cultural humility, 73

culturally sensitive approaches: for in-session work, 59. *See also* diverse clients

cultural-sensitive therapy, 2; Stages of Change model and, 10–11. *See also* diverse clients

cyclical psychodynamic psychotherapy, 1

Dalai Lama, 62–63, 93, 131

daydreaming, 169

DBT. *See* dialectical behavioral therapy

decisional balance exercise. *See* cost-benefit analysis

deep diaphragmatic breathing, 8; as body work, 59; in-session work and, 58–59

deliberate practice, 1

demandingness, 135

dementia, 166
Depakote, 165
depression. *See* major depressive disorders
*Diagnostic Statistical Manual of Mental
    Disorders*: *3rd Edition (DSM-III)*, alcohol
    abuse in, 15; *5th Edition (DSM-V)*, 32–33
dialectical behavioral therapy (DBT), 1;
    radical acceptance in, 90; relationship with
    clients in, 20; unconditional life acceptance,
    87; unconditional other acceptance, 87;
    unconditional self-acceptance, 87
DIBS. *See* disputing irrational beliefs
DID. *See* dissociative identity disorder
DiGiuseppe, Ray, 35
discomfort tolerance, 136
discounting of positive events, 136
discovery method, 157
disputing irrational beliefs (DIBS), 136–37
dissociative identity disorder (DID), 150
diverse clients: active listening with, 75; adverse
    childhood events and, 71; under Americans
    with Disabilities Act, 72–73; cognitive
    behavioral theory and, 72; consultation *versus*
    therapy approaches, 77; cultural humility and,
    73; diversity, equity, and inclusion strategies,
    72; "Do No Harm" principle and, 74; foreign
    films as research source for, 77; insurance
    strategies for, 180–81; meditation and, 73–74;
    microaggressions and, 74–75; motivational
    interviewing with, 75; neurodivergent
    acceptance for, 75, 77; poverty influences on,
    71–72; racism and, 71–72; rejection of self-
    blame, 74; religious beliefs and faith of, 72,
    76; self-reflection for counselors, 73–74
diversity, equity, and inclusion strategies, 72
"Do No Harm" principle, 74
dopamine deficiency, MDD and, 113–14
Doyle, Kristene, 175
dream analysis, 130–31
The Drunkard's Walk (Mlodinow), 91
Dryden, Wendy, 31
*DSM-III. See Diagnostic Statistical Manual of
    Mental Disorders, 3rd Edition*
*DSM-V. See Diagnostic Statistical Manual of
    Mental Disorders, 5th Edition*
Dweck, Carol, 149
Dworkin, Andrea, 151
dysthymia. *See* persistent depressive disorder

EBCT. *See* exposure-based cognitive therapy
ECT. *See* electroconvulsive therapy
Edison, Thomas, 70

EET. *See* empathy and encouragement therapy
EFT. *See* emotion focused therapy
ego, 146
Ehrenreich, Barbara, 98
electroconvulsive therapy (ECT), 171
Ellis, Albert: ABC(DE) exercises, vii, 31, 51–55;
    Buddhism and, 19; cognitive behavioral
    therapy, vii, 11–12; personal background,
    53; rational emotive therapy, vii, 11; rational
    therapy and, 11; unconditional life acceptance,
    87; unconditional other acceptance, 87;
    unconditional self-acceptance, 87; vital
    absorbing creative interest approach, 171–72
EMDR. *See* eye movement desensitization and
    reprocessing
emotional goals, of therapy, 40–41
emotional reasoning, 136
emotion focused therapy (EFT), 1, 12, 97
emotion regulation therapy (ERT), 1
emotions, feelings and: chairwork and, 107; goal-
    setting for, 99; identification and labeling of,
    98–99; negative, 99; over-emoting, 97–98;
    under-emoting, 97–98
empathy, 25
empathy and encouragement therapy (EET), 49
enteric nervous system, 115
Epictetus, 11, 42, 63
Epicurus, 42
Erickson, Milton, 13
ERP. *See* exposure and response prevention
ERT. *See* emotion regulation therapy
ethics, in initial assessment approaches, 33–34
eulogies, 120
executive coaching, 161
exercise: between-session work and, 70; as
    nonmedical alternative, 170
existential beliefs, therapeutic goals influenced
    by, 43–44
existential psychotherapy, 1
expectations, of clients, relationship with clients
    influenced by, 21
experiential avoidance: between-session
    work and, 64–65; if-then statements, 65;
    implementation intentions and, 64; low
    frustration tolerance and, 64; Pomodoro
    Technique, 65
exposure and response prevention (ERP), 1
exposure-based cognitive therapy (EBCT), 1
exposure therapy, 128
eye movement desensitization and reprocessing
    (EMDR), 1, 128

faith, for diverse clients, 72, 76. *See also* spirituality
family therapy, 1
FAP. *See* functional analytic psychotherapy
fate, as concept, 91–92
FDI approach to change. *See* frequency, duration, and intensity approach to change
FDT. *See* future-directed therapy
feedback, in motivational interviewing, 24
feedback loops, 12–13; between-session work and, 67; depression and, 16; panic attacks and, 14, 16; positive, 16; time and, 16
feed-forward loops, 12
feminist theory, 151
feminist therapy, 1
fentanyl, 167
Fils-Aimé, Lyrica, 151
first three memories exercise, 129–30
flash crash, 118
Forecast (Buchanan), 15
fortune, as concept, 91–92
FOT. *See* future-oriented therapy
Frankl, Victor, 44, 120. *See also* logotherapy
free association, 128–29
Freimuth, Marilyn, 36
frequency, duration, and intensity (FDI) approach to change, 118
Freud, Sigmund, theories of: critiques of, 89; lack of scientific evidence for, 13; original seduction theory, 13
friendship, with clients, 23
Fromm, Erich, 99
functional analytic psychotherapy (FAP), 1
future-directed therapy (FDT), 1
future-oriented therapy (FOT), 1, 39

Gafori, Haleh Liza, 100
Gehry, Frank, 178
genetics, 110; alcohol misuse and, 111; for anxiety disorders, 111; attention deficit and hyperactivity disorder and, 111–12; for bipolar disorder, 111
George, David F., 156
Gershon, Michael, 115
Gestalt therapy, 1, 106
Gestalt Therapy Verbatim, 131
Get Out of Your Mind & Into Your Life (Hayes), 20, 103
Glasser, William, 41, 130, 137–38
goals, of therapy: assessment of, 84–85; behavioral, 40; cognitive, 42; drives and, 44–45; emotional, 40–41; existential, 43–44;

interpersonal, 41–42; mindfulness as element of, 41; needs and, 44–45; physical, 42–43; in PRIME theory, 13; relationship-building with clients, 81; Rogerian approach to, 84; sensory, 42–43; of sessions, 23; spiritual, 43–44; thinking, 42
Goldfried, Marvin, 7
Gordon, Judith, 117
graduated exercise therapy, 1
Graham, Carol, 53
gratefulness, mindfulness and, 98
Greenberg, Les, 12, 97, 106
group therapy, 59; individual therapy compared to, 178
grudgingness, 93
guilt, shame as distinct from, 100

habits, in PRIME theory, 12
Hacking, Ian, 150
harm minimization, in initial assessment approaches, 33–34
harm reduction therapy, 1
HARPS. *See* high alcohol recovery persons
Hayes, Steve, 20, 64, 103
Headspace app, 63, 103
helpful/rational beliefs, 53
heroin addiction, 167
Hidden Addiction (Freimuth), 36
Hierarchy of Values exercise (HOV exercise), 92–93, 122
high alcohol recovery persons (HARPS), 21
homework, between-session work as, viii
Horney, Karen, 89, 154
HOV exercise. *See* Hierarchy of Values exercise
Howe, Florence, 151
How to Think More about Sex (Botton), 44
Hula Hoop technique, 91
humanistic therapy, 1
Hurley, Wilson, 63

ICD-10. *See* International Classification of Diseases, 10th Edition
id, 146
identities: clarification of, 150–51; for clients, 146–47; dissociative identity disorder, 150; ego, 146; id, 146; Rogers on, 150; superego, 146; tripartite model for, 146
IFS. *See* Internal Family Systems
if-then statements, 65
imagery, use of: in cognitive behavioral therapy (CBT), 100, 102–3; guided, 102; inference

chaining and, 101–2; rational emotive imagery, 105–6
Imagery Rescripting (ImR), 107
implementation intentions: experiential avoidance and, 64; for in-session work, 49
ImR. *See* Imagery Rescripting
inequity, 151–52
inference chaining, vii, 101–2
initial assessment. *See* assessment
injustice, 151–52
in-session work: ABC(DE) model, 51–55; acceptance and commitment therapy and, 55; assessment instruments for, 82; blaming in, 50; culturally-sensitive approaches to, 59; deep diaphragmatic breathing and, 58–59; defusion of beliefs during, 55, 57; empathy and encouragement therapy and, 49; evaluations of, 57–58; identification of "brain lies," 50–51; implementation intentions for, 49; interpretations of, 57–58; judgment of, 58; managed perceptions of, 57–58; outcome assessment for, 82; rating of, 58; shaming in, 50. *See also* between-session work
insurance, for initial assessment, 34
integrative therapy, 1
Internal Family Systems (IFS), 1
International Classification of Diseases, 10th Edition (ICD-10), 32–33
interpersonal goals, of therapy, 41–42
interpersonal psychotherapy, 2
intersectionality: classism and, 151–52, 156; definition and scope of, 149; development of term, 149; elements of, 149–50; feminist theory and, 151; inequity and, 151–52; injustice and, 151–52; pluralist perspectives and, 152–53; racism and, 151–52, 156; unconscious bias and, 156
interviewing, interviews and. *See* cultural formulation interview; motivational interviewing
irrational beliefs: disputing irrational beliefs, 136–37. *See* unhelpful/irrational beliefs

Jackson, James, 13
James, William, 43, 147, 160
Jung, Carl, 13
Jungian therapy, 2

Kagan, Jerome, 110
Kaptchuk, Ted, 163
KAT. *See* ketamine assisted therapy
Kellogg, Scott, 91, 107

ketamine assisted therapy (KAT), 168
King, Albert, 21
Klonopin, 59
van der Kolk, Bessel, 115
Korzybski, Alfred, 146–47, 156
Kripalu, vii

labeling, 136
Lazarus, Arnold, 30. *See also* multimodal therapy
Leake, George, 21
LFT. *See* low frustration tolerance
life coaching, 161
Lifetrack therapy, 2
Linehan, Marsha, 20, 39; development of mindfulness as modality, 87; religious transformation for, 145. *See also* dialectical behavioral therapy
listening approaches: active listening, 25, 75; nonjudgmental, 126; reflective listening, 25
logotherapy, 2, 44
long-term psychotherapy, 178–79
low frustration distress, 136
low frustration tolerance (LFT), 64

Maguire, Eleanor, 114
major depressive disorders (MDD): Beck Depression Scale, 30; case study for, 182–83; dopamine deficiency and, 113–14; genetic inheritance of, 111; initial assessment for, 35–36; persistent depressive disorder, 56
Man's Search for Meaning (Frankl), 120
Marcus Aurelius, 11
marital counseling: initial assessment for, 34; ₅slow discussions, 159–60
Marlatt, Alan, 117
Maslow's Hierarchy of Needs, 44
Maultsby, Maxie, 105
May, Rollo, 9
MBCT. *See* mindfulness-based cognitive therapy
MBSR. *See* mindfulness-based stress reduction
McDonald, Michele, 89
MDD. *See* major depressive disorders
MDMA use, 168
medical model, of psychotherapy, 12. *See also* neurochemical model
medications, therapeutic: advantages of, 164–65; advertising for, 163; for attention deficit and hyperactivity disorder, 164–65; atypical antipsychotics, 166; in combined therapies, 171–72; critiques of, 163–64; for dementia, 166; disadvantages of, 164–65; internists and, 165; ketamine assisted therapy, 168;

norepinephrine and dopamine reuptake inhibitors, 114; overutilized, 166–67; placebo effect and, 163–64; placebo study and, 163; in psychedelic-assisted therapy, 168; psychiatrists and, 165–66; psychopharmacologists and, 165–66; for schizophrenia, 166; selective serotonin re-uptake inhibitors, 59, 164; serotonin and norepinephrine reuptake inhibitors, 59; underutilized, 167–68. *See also* nonmedical approaches; *specific medications*

meditation, 59; as between-session work, 62–63; diverse clients and, 73–74; as nonmedical approach, 170; therapeutic approaches to, 163–72

MET. *See* motivational enhancement therapy

metabolic syndrome (MetS), 166

metastability, 15; mindfulness and, 88; neural modular networks and, 14; teaching about, 119

methadone, 167

MetS. *See* metabolic syndrome

MI. *See* motivational interviewing

microaggressions, 74–75

Miller, George, 105

Miller, William, 10, 23–24. *See also* motivational interviewing

mindfulness: CALM app, 63, 103; client acceptance and, 88–91; Columbo Technique and, 94–96; compassion and, 98; development as treatment modality, 87; as goal of therapy, 41; gratefulness and, 98; grudgingness and, 93; Headspace app, 63, 103; Hierarchy of Values exercise, 92–93; Hula Hoop technique, 91; metastability and, 88; mind-wandering, 93–94; RAIN technique, 89, 100; shoulding and, 89–90; willingness and, 93

mindfulness-based cognitive therapy (MBCT), 2

mindfulness-based stress reduction (MBSR), 2

mind-wandering, 93–94

Miracle Question, 56

Mischel, Walter, 4

Mlodinow, Leonard, 91

motivation, for therapy, for clients, 20

motivational enhancement therapy (MET), 2

motivational interviewing (MI), 2; active listening as part of, 25; change talk in, 25; closed-ended questions in, 25; cognitive defusion techniques, 120; DEARS in, 24; with diverse clients, 75; feedback in, 24; FRAME, 24; Miller and, 10; OARS in, 24–25; reflective listening as part of, 25; relationship with clients and, 23–25; self-assessment instruments in, 24; unhelpful beliefs, 119–20

Mounjaro. *See* tirzepatide

multicultural therapy, 2

multimodal therapy, 2, 30; imagery use in, 100, 102–3

multisystemic therapy, 2

Myers & Briggs personality tests, 147

NAFLD. *See* nonalcoholic fatty liver disease

Naloxone, 167

Naltrexone, 167

narrative therapy, 2

NDRIs. *See* norepinephrine and dopamine reuptake inhibitors

needs: goals of therapy influenced by, 44–45; Maslow's Hierarchy of Needs, 44

negative emotions, 99

negative exaggeration, 135

negative feedback loops, 67

Neisser, Ulric, 11

neural modular networks, 16; metastability and, 14; neuroplasticity, 114–15

neurochemical model, 12, 113, 116

neurodivergence, acceptance of by culturally diverse clients, 75, 77

New York Times, viii

Niebuhr, Reinold, 90

nonalcoholic fatty liver disease (NAFLD), 166

nondirective psychotherapy, 47

nonjudgmental listening, 126

nonmedical approaches, 168–71, *169*

norepinephrine and dopamine reuptake inhibitors (NDRIs), 114

NOS assessment. *See* not otherwise specified

note-taking, 20–22

not otherwise specified (NOS assessment), 32

obituaries, 120

Odyssey (Wilson), 109

Omega Institute, vii

OQ-45. *See* Outcome Questionnaire 45

original seduction theory, adverse childhood events study and, 13

ORS. *See* Outcome Rating Scale

Outcome Questionnaire 45 (OQ-45), 30, 82

Outcome Rating Scale (ORS), 82

overeating, as behavioral problem, viii

over-emoting, 97–98

overgeneralizing, 136

Ozempic. *See* semaglutide

Padesky, Christine, 31–32, 151

panic attacks: between-session work for, 66–67; factors for, 14; feedback loops and, 14, 16; positive feedback loops and, 16
Paxil, 59
PCL-5 Scale, 30
PDD. *See* persistent depressive disorder
peer rejection, 66
Perls, Fritz, 9, 106–7, 131
persistent depressive disorder (PDD), 56
personality: borderline personality disorder, 149; character compared to, 147, 149; Myers & Briggs personality tests, 147
personalizing, 136
person-centered therapy, 2
physicalizing, 103, 105
placebo effect, 163–64
placebo study, 163
polyvagal theory, 13
Pomodoro Technique, 65
positive feedback loops, panic attacks and, 16
positive psychotherapy, 2
posttraumatic growth, 131
post-traumatic stress disorder (PTSD), 107; cognitive processing therapy for, 126–27; complex post-traumatic stress disorder, 125–26; exposure therapy for, 128
poverty, 71–72
prayer: between-session work and, 62–63; Serenity Prayer, 90
pre-contemplation stage, in Stages of Change model, 10
preparation stage, in Stages of Change model, 10
PRIME model/theory: conditioning/habits in, 12; evaluations in, 12; external factors in, 12; feedback loops, 12–13; feed-forward loops, 12; goals in, 13; goals of therapy and, 13; for initial assessment, 32–33; internal factors in, 12; plans in, 13; responses in, 12
protective behavioral strategies, 121
Prozac, 12
psychedelic-assisted therapy, 168
psychiatrists, 165–66
PSYCHLOPS. *See* Psychological Outcomes Profiles Questionnaire
psychoanalysis, 2; relationship with clients and, 27; as top-down model, 61; transference between client and counselor, 27
psychodynamic psychotherapy, 2
Psychological Outcomes Profiles Questionnaire (PSYCHLOPS), 82
psychopharmacologists, 165–66
psychopharmacotherapy, 2

psychotherapy: alternative therapies, viii; bottom-up model for, 43, 47; brain disease model, viii; coaching compared to, 157–59; collaborative approaches to, viii, 7–9; as future-oriented, viii; as goal-oriented, viii; historical developments in, viii; integrative approaches to, 4; long-term, 178–79; methodological approach to, 5; nondirective, 47; popularity of specific schools, 5; short-term, 178–79; top-down model for, 43. *See also* medications; research; *specific therapies*; *specific topics*
PTSD. *See* post-traumatic stress disorder
Purposive Behavior in Animals and Men (Tolman), 39

quantum change, in Stages of Change model, 10–11

racism, 71–72; intersectionality and, 151–52, 156
radical acceptance, 90; between-session work and, 140
RAIN technique, 89, 100, 177–78
randomness concept, 91–92
Rating of Outcome Scale (ROS), 82
rational beliefs. *See* helpful/rational beliefs
rational emotive behavior therapy (REBT), 2, 51; with bipolar disorder, 26; historical development of, 11
rational emotive imagery (REI), 105–6
rational emotive therapy (RET), vii, 11
rational therapy (RT), 11
reality shifting, 170
reality therapy, 2, 137
REBT. *See* rational emotive behavior therapy
reflective listening, 25
REI. *See* rational emotive imagery
relapse prevention, 2
Relapse Prevention (Marlatt and Gordon), 117
relationship with clients: in acceptance and commitment therapy, 20; burnout and, 21; counselor expectations of clients and, 21; counselor self-care influenced by, 21; in dialectical behavioral therapy, 20; empathy as element in, 25; friendship conflicts in, 23; helpfulness element in, 25; with high alcohol recovery persons, 21; motivational interviewing and, 23–25; normalization of, 22–23; note-taking during session, 20–22; personal opinions about clients as factor in, 21; personal self-disclosures and, 21, 27–28;

psychoanalytic theory and, 27; session goals, 23; transference in, 27

religious beliefs: for diverse clients, 72, 76; as nonmedical alternative, 169. *See also* spirituality

repressed memories, 130

research, on psychotherapeutic approaches, advantages of, 6

Resick, Patricia, 126–27, 135

resistance, 118; to collaboration, 8

RET. *See* rational emotive therapy

risk-taking exercises, 63–64

Robb, Hank, 93

Rogers, Carl, 9, 43; on agenda setting for therapy, 47; client-centered therapy, 1, 47; on goals of therapy, 84; on identity, 150; nonjudgmental listening, 126; unconditional regard, 151

role-playing, 160

ROS. *See* Rating of Outcome Scale

RT. *See* rational therapy

Russell, Bertrand, 11

SAD. *See* seasonal affective disorder

Saks, Elyn, viii

Santos, Laurie, 50, 89

schema therapy, 2

schizophrenia, 166

seasonal affective disorder (SAD), 170

The Second Brain (Gershon), 115

selective serotonin re-uptake inhibitors (SSRIs), 59, 164

the self, 146; transcendental self, 115–16; unitary, 147

self-assessment, in motivational interviewing, 24

self-care, for counselors, 21

self-compassion, 116

self-confidence, strategies for, 153–54

self-criticism, 156

self-disclosures, by counselors, 21, 27–28

self-downing, 136

self-examination therapy, 2

self-help models, viii

self-pity, 156

self-system psychotherapy, 2

semaglutide, 168

Serenity Prayer, 90

serotonin and norepinephrine reuptake inhibitors (SNRIs), 59

shame, shaming and: attention deficit and hyperactivity disorder and, 112; guilt as distinct from, 100; in-session work and, 50

shame attacks, 100

Shapiro, Francine, 128

shell shock, 124

short-term psychotherapy, 178–79

shoulding, 89–90

sleep habits, 116; between-session work and, 69–70

sleep hygiene, 170

slow discussions, 159–60

small talk, in initial assessment, 30

smartphones, between-session work and, 69–70

SMART Recovery groups, 59, 171, 174

SNRIs. *See* serotonin and norepinephrine reuptake inhibitors

Socratic questioning, 54, 127

solution-focused brief therapy, 2; Miracle Question in, 56

spirituality: goals of therapy influenced by, 43–44. *See also* prayer

SSRIs. *See* selective serotonin re-uptake inhibitors

Stages of Change model, 118–19; action stage, 10; for alcohol abuse, 37; between-session work and, 61; contemplation stage, 10; critiques of, 10–11; cultural limitations of, 10–11; in initial assessment, 30–31; positive aspects of, 10; pre-contemplation stage, 10; preparation stage, 10; quantum change in, 10

Stoicism, 11, 63

stress management, as behavioral problem, viii

suicidal ideation, between-session work as positive influence on, 66

sun therapy, 170

superego, 146

systemic therapy, 2

take-home therapy exercises, 65

Talks for Teachers (James), 147

talk therapy, 164

telehealth, 179

termination of clients, 181

three-column technique, 138–39

tirzepatide, 168

TMS. *See* transcranial magnetic stimulation

Tolman, Edward C., 39

TOP. *See* Treatment Outcome Package

transactional analysis, 2

transcendentalism, 43; brain development and, 115–16

transcranial magnetic stimulation (TMS), 171

transdiagnostic analysis, 2

transdiagnostic CBT, 2

transference, between client and counselor, 27

Transformational Chairwork (Kellogg), 107
transtheoretical model (TTM), 10–11. *See also*
 Stages of Change model
trauma-informed counseling and therapy, shaming
 as cultural response, 124
trauma recovery and empowerment model, 2
trauma theory, 13
Treatment Outcome Package (TOP), 177
TTM. *See* transtheoretical model
Tutu, Desmond, 62–63, 93

unconditional life acceptance (ULA), 87
unconditional other acceptance (UOA), 87
unconditional regard, 151
unconditional self-acceptance (USA), 87
unconscious bias, 156
Unconscious Bias (George), 156
under-emoting, 97–98
unhelpful beliefs, 53, 119–20, 136–37
unhelpful/irrational beliefs, 53
unified protocol, 2
unitary self, 147
UOA. *See* unconditional other acceptance

USA. *See* unconditional self-acceptance

VACI approach. *See* vital absorbing creative
 interest approach
value clarification exercises, 139–40
varenicline, 168
Veterans Administration CBT program, 30
Vispassana Hawai'i, 89
vital absorbing creative interest approach (VACI
 approach), 171–72

Watters, Ethan, 71
wearable technology, between-session work and,
 69–70
Wellbutrin, 114
West, Robert, 153
What Should I Do with My Life (Bronson), 120
Wilson, Emily, 109

Xanax, 59

Zoloft, 59
Zyban. *See* bupropion

About the Author

F. Michler Bishop, PhD, is in private practice in New York City after retiring from the Albert Ellis Institute (AEI), where he worked closely with Dr. Ellis for more than 20 years, running groups and workshops. During his long career, he has advocated for a compassionate, goal-focused modern therapeutic approach, integrating a variety of research-based treatment options with alternative healing techniques and activities that a client has found helpful in the past. The overall objective is to create a unique therapy for each client. As one of the founders of SMART Recovery®, he was instrumental in the development of SMART Recovery's growth and its Four-Point Program. He has conducted numerous workshops on CBT, rational emotive behavior therapy (REBT), MI, and SMART Recovery in the United States and internationally. He worked at AEI for more than 35 years, seeing clients with a wide variety of problems, including anxiety and mood disorders, impulse control, and relationship issues.

www.ingramcontent.com/pod-product-compliance
Lightning Source LLC
Chambersburg PA
CBHW080132270326
41926CB00021B/4451